SECRET WALKS

A WALKING GUIDE
TO THE
HIDDEN TRAILS
OF LOS ANGELES

SANTA
MONICA
PRESS

Published by:

Santa Monica Press LLC
P.O. Box 850
Solana Beach, CA 92075
1-800-784-9553
www.santamonicapress.com
books@santamonicapress.com

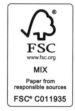

FSC
www.fsc.org
MIX
Paper from
responsible sources
FSC® C011935

Printed in the United States

Santa Monica Press books are available at special quantity discounts
when purchased in bulk by corporations, organizations, or groups.
Please call our Special Sales department at 1-800-784-9553.

This book is intended to provide general information. The publisher, author,
distributor, and copyright owner are not engaged in rendering professional
advice or services. The publisher, author, distributor, and copyright owner
are not liable or responsible to any person or group with respect to any loss,
illness, or injury caused or alleged to be caused by the information found in
this book.

ISBN-13 978-1-59580-082-4

Library of Congress Cataloging-in-Publication Data

Fleming, Charles.
Secret walks : a walking guide to the hidden trails of Los Angeles / Charles
Fleming.
    pages cm
Includes index.
ISBN 978-1-59580-082-4 (paperback)
1. Walking—California—Los Angeles—Guidebooks. 2. Trails—California—Los
Angeles—Guidebooks. 3. Los Angeles (Calif.)—Tours. 4. Los Angeles (Calif.)—
Guidebooks. I. Title.
F869.L83F586 2015
917.94'940453—dc23
                    2014045520

Cover and interior design and production by Future Studio
Cover illustration and maps by Bryan Duddles
Photos by Charles Fleming

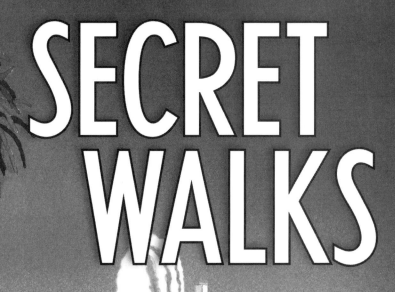

SECRET WALKS

A WALKING GUIDE TO THE HIDDEN TRAILS OF LOS ANGELES

CHARLES FLEMING

AUTHOR OF *SECRET STAIRS*

CONTENTS

PART FIVE: EAST LOS ANGELES

PART SIX: PASADENA & ENVIRONS

PART SEVEN: SAN FERNANDO VALLEY & ENVIRONS

PART EIGHT: WEST LOS ANGELES & BEACHES

PART NINE: SOUTH BAY

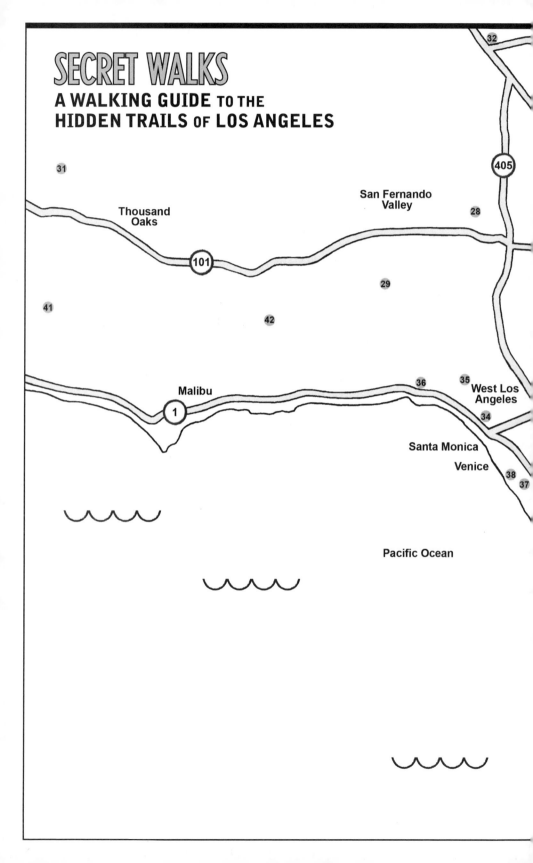

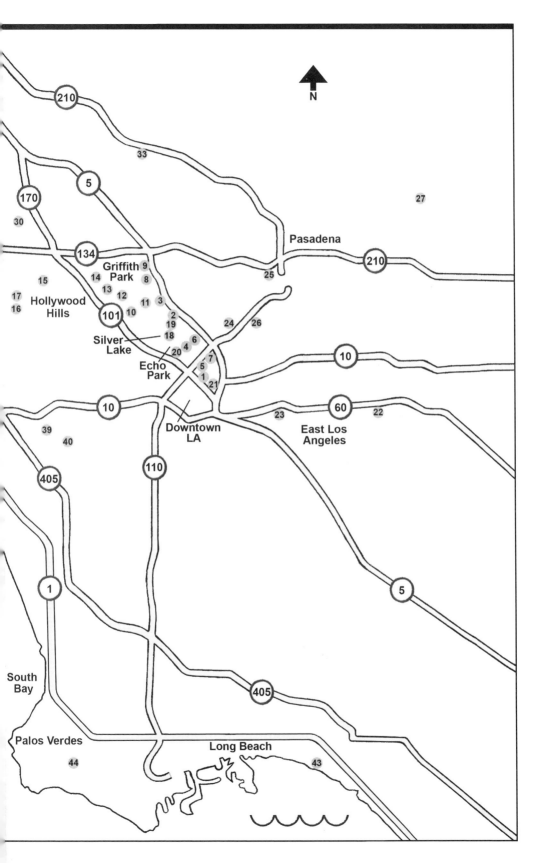

INTRODUCTION

In 2005, I was scheduled for a back operation. I'd already had two complete hip replacements. I'd already had two spinal surgeries. This was to be my third, in three years. And I couldn't face it. The prospect of another hospital stay, another surgery, and another rehab was just overwhelming.

So I canceled the surgery date. I decided to try something different.

I decided to try walking.

Even though I was in terrible pain and couldn't work or drive, I'd found that if I could get on my feet and move, I felt a little better.

So I started walking. I went a single block the first day. I went two blocks the second day. I went a little farther the third. I walked all that week. I felt better. So I kept walking.

When I felt stronger, I included some elevation. I started climbing the steeper streets around my house in Silver Lake. To keep it interesting, I started exploring the public stairways that laced the hills here. I resolved to plot out circular walks linking them together, for no other reason than to keep me walking.

Those rudimentary circular walks became *Secret Stairs: A Walking Guide to the Historic Staircases of Los Angeles*, published in 2010, and *Secret Stairs East Bay: A Walking Guide to the Historic Staircases of Berkeley and Oakland*, published two years later.

By then, I was healthy again. I never did show up for that third back surgery. I started playing tennis again. I took up snowboarding, and bought a motorcycle and began riding the trails and deserts again, for the first time in decades.

As long as I kept walking, I kept feeling good. So I walked every day. To support the books, I began leading a free monthly stair walk, which soon was drawing sixty to a hundred eager stair explorers. Later, I got an offer to write the L.A. Walks column for the *Los Angeles Times*, and ended up working there full-time.

As time passed and I designed more walks and met more walkers, it became evident that there were all kinds of people who wanted to walk, but couldn't manage the stairs—elderly people, parents with young children in strollers, and people who were out of shape or recovering from injuries or surgeries.

From this, the idea for *Secret Walks* was born. This is a collection of walks that *anyone* can do. Many are under two miles. Many are flat, with virtually no elevation change at all. Many can be done by someone using a wheelchair, or a family pushing a stroller. And they're all great places to visit—interesting, little-known, hidden gems that will enhance anyone's appreciation of the city.

A reader familiar with hiking in the Los Angeles area might study the table of contents and conclude that I have left out many of the region's most popular walks. That's because I have. Early on, I decided there was no need to chronicle local hikes that are already well-known. So you won't find Runyon Canyon, or Temescal Gateway Park, or Malibu Creek State Park here.

Those walks have already been covered in other guidebooks, and are already so well-established that they're crowded.

These walks are the ones most people aren't already walking.

The litmus test was simple: if they were great walks that I had never walked or heard about, they were candidates for inclusion in this book.

There was great pleasure in determining which walks to include. As was the case with both *Secret Stairs* books, gathering the information for this collection gave me a mandate to investigate parks, canyons, and corners of the city that I'd always known about but never explored.

Some walks were familiar to me from years gone by—like

Griffith Park's Fern Dell, which my daughters loved when they were young. Some were familiar to me because I'd heard about them or had seen them from afar, like the giant steps at Baldwin Hills Scenic Overlook, or the Naples Canals in Long Beach.

But others were brand new. I found Peanut Lake just by looking at a map. Lovely! A friend told me about Paradise Falls. Fantastic!

All of them were near at hand, very few required much of a drive, and almost all were easily accessible by public transport (for these criteria were part of the litmus test, too). Except for a few instances where there is a fee for weekend parking, all of the walks are open to the public, free of charge.

I had low expectations when the first *Secret Stairs* book was published. During the years I spent finding the hidden stairs, mapping them, and designing the walks, I encountered almost no one. The stairs really felt secret.

But in the years since, I have continued to be surprised and delighted by the book's popularity and by the literally hundreds of people who have told me how much the book has meant to them. Some have told me how they got fit, lost weight, and began dating for the first time in years. A few have told me how they met a new friend, or a new partner, on the monthly stair walks. Dozens of people have said variations of, "I have lived here for thirty years, and I never even knew this place existed."

And many of them have told me that they had the same experience I did in the making of *Secret Stairs*—that exploring Los Angeles on these urban trails changed their lives and their feelings about living in this sometimes difficult city.

I hope this collection of walks will have a similar impact, and introduce residents and visitors to parts of Los Angeles they wouldn't otherwise encounter, and help them fall in love with Los Angeles in ways that may surprise them.

Each of the forty-four walks in this book is rated for distance, duration, and difficulty on a scale of one to five, with five being most difficult compared to the other walks in this book. The measurements are all estimated. A fit person will have no difficulty at all with a five. A fast walker or a hiker in a hurry will be able to complete the loops faster than I did. A slow walker, really soaking it all in, might find that a forty-five-minute walk takes an hour.

There isn't, however, a way to measure joy and pleasure. I hope those using this book find as much value in it as I have while preparing it.

Map Legend

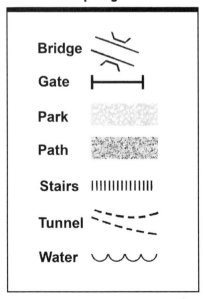

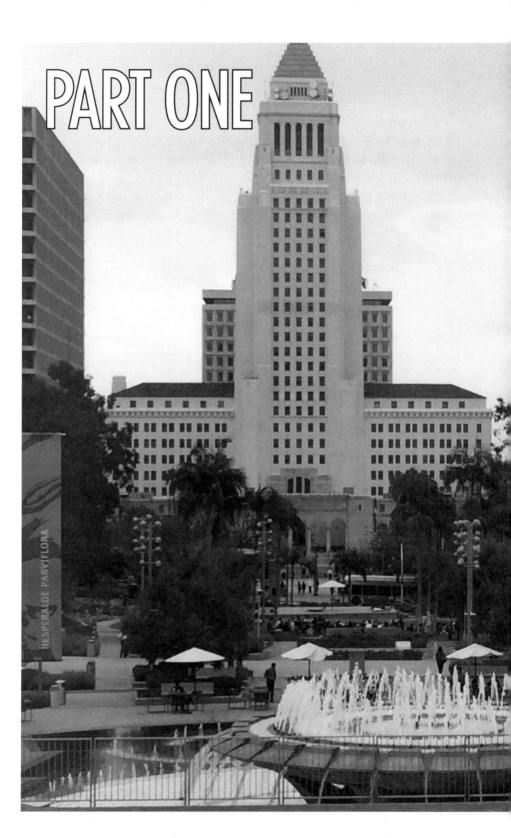

PART ONE

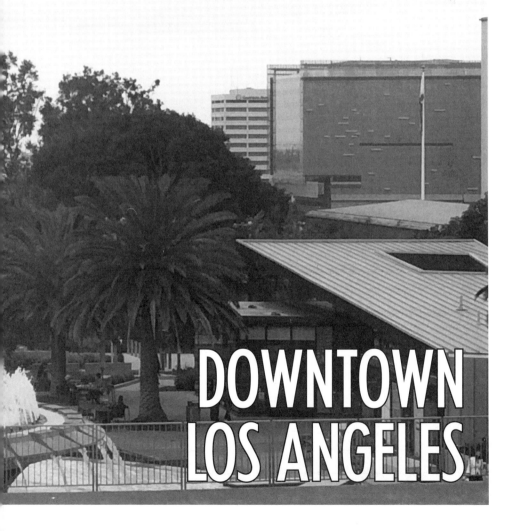

DOWNTOWN LOS ANGELES

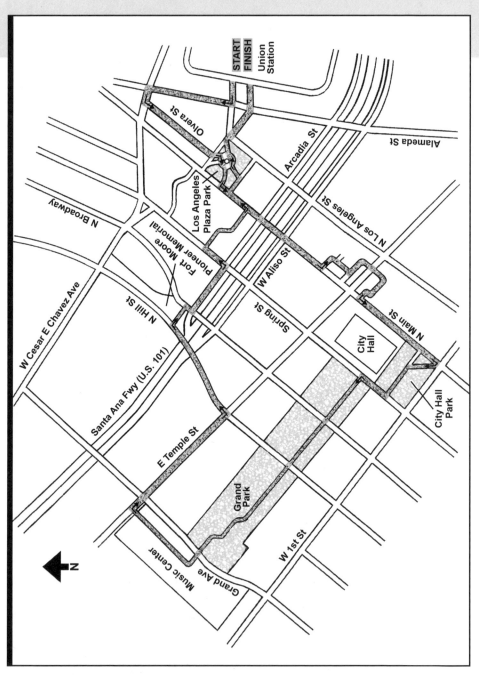

Overleaf: A view of Grand Park and City Hall from downtown L.A.'s Music Center.

WALK #1

DOWNTOWN L.A. HISTORY WALK
DISTANCE: **2.75 miles**
DIFFICULTY: **2**
DURATION: **1 hour 30 minutes**
DETAILS: **Free and metered street parking. Dogs on leash allowed. Metro buses #4, #10, #40, and #442.**

This is a walk through history, starting with Los Angeles's roots and concluding with its newest city park and biggest downtown cathedral.

Begin this journey at Union Station on Alameda Street, near the heart of L.A.'s historic center. Before starting the walk, take some time to enjoy the station. Once a dominant feature of the city skyline, its exterior was often the cinematic establishing shot that told audiences they were in L.A. The interior has a lot to see. Admire the beamed, hand-painted ceilings, marble floors, cork walls, brass fittings, and leather seats. There are places to eat and drink here, too, from the high-end Traxx restaurant and bar located at the front of the station to the lower-end snacks further inside.

Across the breezeway, check out the once-bustling restaurant space that used to be a Harvey House, one of the many restaurants operated by businessman Fred Harvey in the early railroad days in stations across the West. The space is now home to the Imperial Western Brewing Company.

Also, don't miss the main ticket counter area, which is no longer in use. If it looks familiar, that's because it is frequently used in movies and TV shows.

Leave the station through its original main entrance, heading west. Follow the sidewalk to Alameda Street and turn right. Walk to the corner at Cesar E. Chavez Avenue, and turn left to cross Alameda. Once on the other side, turn left again, into Olvera Street.

This is Los Angeles's tribute to its Mexican roots—a block of "authentic" Mexican shops and restaurants that isn't really authentic at all. Although the block contains what is said to be the city's oldest house—the Avila Adobe, built in 1818—the street itself, and all its shops and "Mexican" flavor, were the invention of local doyenne Christine Sterling, who sought to restore the street to its imaginary Mexican origins. (It does, in fact, have old Mexican roots. Agustin Olvera was an early Los Angeles judge, and Francisco Avila was an early city mayor.) Using prison labor and donations from citizens like *Los Angeles Times* publisher Harry Chandler, Sterling oversaw the 1928 construction of Olvera Street, which has remained more or less intact ever since.

Enjoy the ficus and pepper tree shade as you walk up the lone block, filled with the scents of tanned leather, fresh tortillas, and toys and trinkets made from Chinese plastic. At the top of the street, you'll find Los Angeles Plaza Park. Under a massive shade tree is a fine bandstand that often hosts musical events. Circle around the back of the bandstand, then bend right, aiming for the stretch of North Main Street that runs between Pico House on your left and the Garnier and Brunswig buildings on your right.

This is more old city history. Pico House was a luxury hotel, built in 1869 by Pio Pico, the last Mexican governor of the territory of Southern California, who used the architect that designed the Cathedral of Saint Vibiana. The Garnier and Brunswig buildings, both from the 1880s, were also important early structures for the growing metropolis.

Continue south on Main, past Pico House, and past the big

black-and-white historic pictures inside the Plaza de Cultura y Artes building. Cross Arcadia Street, cross over the Santa Ana Freeway (U.S. 101), and then cross Aliso Street. As you go, admire the lovely City Hall building rising before you. Even more than Union Station, it was the identifying feature of the Los Angeles landscape, and should be familiar to anyone who has ever watched movies shot from the 1930s to the 1960s. Continue half a block, then turn in to the small park on your left.

The large, three-legged beast in the plaza is what's left of the Triforium. Built in 1975, this sixty-foot-tall whimsy was meant to sense the presence of pedestrians below and perform for them, using music played on a carillion of seventy-nine glass bells and a light show displayed on stained glass panels. This public artwork had a short life, and has not functioned for many years.

Over to the left, look for a pedestrian bridge, elegantly curved like something from a Japanese garden. Use this to cross Temple Street. On the other side, walk under some feeble trees and return to Main Street, turning left at the sidewalk. (Down below you, incidentally, is the Los Angeles Mall, a subterranean street of shops and restaurants that, though open during the week, go dark during most of the weekend.)

At First Street, turn right and cross Main Street, then bear right into City Hall Park, the grounds surrounding the seat of the Los Angeles government. City Hall is iconic, and it's phallic, and it's still a fine building. At the time of its construction in 1928, it rose to 452 feet—the first high rise in Southern California and, until 1964, the tallest building in the city. (The Union Bank Plaza on Figueroa, which stands 516 feet tall, stole that crown when it was completed.)

Enjoy the grounds and the views from the park to the stark new Los Angeles Police Department headquarters across First Street and the stately old *Los Angeles Times* building—although the newspaper no longer occupies the building—across Spring Street. When you get to Spring, bear right, walking slightly uphill. At the pedestrian crossing, cross Spring and enter Grand Park.

This is Los Angeles's newest big urban green space. It stretches from the front of City Hall, across the equivalent of four long city blocks, and up to the plaza that is home to the Music Center, Ahmanson Theatre, and Mark Taper Forum. Enjoy its wide lawns, secluded shady areas, hot pink seats and benches—all of them free-roaming and untethered, so you can arrange them as you like—and water features. (There's also a Starbucks, located near the top of the park.)

You'll cross Broadway and Hill Street as you go (and Olive Street, or what used to be Olive Street, marked now only by a line of olive trees). Finally you will climb several sets of stairs (there are ramps for those who can't climb stairs) to Grand Avenue. Cross this, and go up a final flight of stairs into the arts plaza.

To the right are the Ahmanson Theatre and the Mark Taper Forum. In the middle of the plaza you'll find a fountain and, usually, some food and beverage carts.

After you've enjoyed all of this, turn toward the Ahmanson and walk all the way to the northern end of the arts plaza. Find a staircase dropping down to the corner of Grand and Temple, kitty-corner from the Cathedral of Our Lady of the Angels. Cross both streets to get to the cathedral.

One of Los Angeles's first churches was the cathedral known as Nuestra Señora la Reina de Los Angeles. The one standing in front you now is the newer American version. Designed by Spanish architect Rafael Moneo and featuring elements (like the bronze doors) from local sculptor Robert Graham, the cathedral was opened with great civic fanfare in 2002, after an expenditure of almost $200 million in construction costs. Among those interred here are Gregory Peck and the remains of Saint Vibiana.

Descending on Temple, go past the cathedral and turn left onto Hill Street. Walk two blocks, again crossing the Santa Ana Freeway. Just beyond this, to your left, is an unusual historic monument. This is what's left of Fort Moore, where in 1846 a small band of U.S. Marines held off an assault by the local Mexicans and Californios, who for some reason resented being ruled by a foreign occupying force. The Marines were expelled, but returned in force. Los Angeles was taken some months later, and has been under U.S. control ever since. The fort was later rebuilt by a platoon of Mormons. All of this strange history is recounted artfully on the remaining walls.

Across Hill Street from this monument, back at the corner of Hill and Arcadia, find the staircase that drops down from Hill Street to Broadway. Then follow the sidewalk to descend another block. Cross Spring Street to the south side of the street, then turn left and walk a half block along Spring.

At a break in the long line of fencing, find the little staircase on your right, and descend to a walkway that runs between the original cathedral of Nuestra Señora la Reina de Los Angeles on your left and the museum known as Plaza de Culturas y Artes on your right—free to the public, and containing some great examples of early California art.

Follow that walkway to Main Street, cross Main, and once more enter the main plaza at the head of Olvera Street. Crossing this, take note from this angle of the area's other church, a 1925 Methodist Church, which has a fine, tiled cupola dome. You will also probably see a forlorn donkey attached to a cart, whose job is to sit underneath or stand next to tourists who want their pictures taken.

Cross the plaza, heading generally toward Union Station and its clock tower. On the left, you'll note a mural depicting the annual Blessing of the Animals (this ceremony does take place here every year on the Saturday before Easter). Also nearby are a statue of Spain's King Carlos III and a huge equestrian statue of Antonio Aguilar, a popular Mexican actor and singer who was one of the first Mexicans to get his star on the Hollywood Walk of Fame.

Drop down a few stairs to Alameda Street. Cross Alameda to the front of Union Station, and you will find yourself back at your starting point.

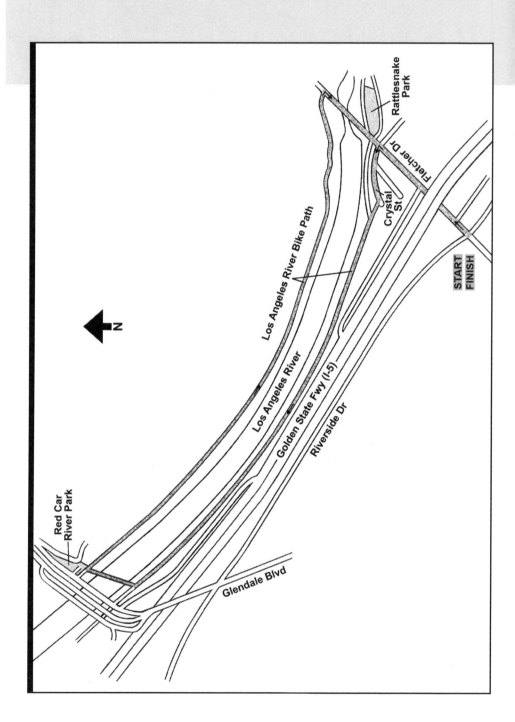

WALK #2

L.A. RIVER WALK SOUTH
DISTANCE: **2.2 miles**
DIFFICULTY: **1**
DURATION: **1 hour**
DETAILS: **Dogs on leash allowed.**
Wheelchair accessible.
Metro buses #96 and #603.

This stretch of the Los Angeles River bank may one day be a fine, green waterside park. For now, it's a good place to stretch your legs, get some fresh air, and see some unusual bird life.

Begin your walk at the intersection of Riverside Drive and Fletcher Drive, perhaps at Rick's Burgers or trendy Salazar just up the road. Head east on Fletcher and pass under the Golden State Freeway (I-5), on the north side of the street. When you get to Crystal Street, turn left and walk to the end of the road—where you'll find the entrance to the Los Angeles River Bike Path, sometimes referred to as the Los Angeles River Greenway Trail. Turn in to the left and begin walking north, with the river on your right.

This section of the river is a prime example of what's happening all along its length: the concrete water sluice, built to control rainwater inundation after Los Angeles saw deadly floods in the early part of the twentieth century, has now begun to take on the features of a natural river.

The flat, clean bike path, which is lighted for evening walks and rides, parallels a green belt largely free of debris and trash. Willow trees have taken root. Rushes and reeds have flourished, as has the bird population. An early morning walk offers views of stilts, herons, egrets, and a variety of ducks.

Walk upstream on the path (being mindful of the bicycles who claim the right of way). As the roar of the freeway softens, look straight ahead for a view of the Griffith Park hills. Far off to the right, you may get a glimpse of the buildings of Forest Lawn's Glendale property, too.

As you approach a complicated series of overpasses, watch for the new pedestrian bridge on your right. This runs along the tracks of the old Red Car line that crossed the river here. Opened in early 2020, it's only for bikes and pedestrians. Enjoy and cross to the opposite bank.

This is Red Car River Park, whose murals tell some of the story of Los Angeles's once-great public transportation system. (A fuller story, though fictional, was told in the book *Who Killed Roger Rabbit?* and the film based on it, *Who Framed Roger Rabbit*.)

Head south along the river, with the water to your right. If it's a dry day, you might stroll down the sloped bank to the flat walkway at the water's edge. Do *not* do this, however, if the river is moving fast, if it's raining, or if it looks like it might start raining. This is a *dry day* exercise only.

At the water's edge, the birds may be quite close—mergansers, great egrets, snowy egrets, osprey, sandpipers, stilts, great blue heron, and green heron are almost always visible. Varieties of fish are said to swim in the river, too, though I've never seen them.

The islands that have formed around the trees in the middle of the river are tempting, and it's hard not think of Huck Finn adventures beginning here. But wading isn't recommended, and the people who may have already made their homes on the island, in the dry season, may not appreciate visitors. Best stick to the bank.

The walk continues on, flat and gentle, at both the river's edge and the pathway the runs along the top of its bank. In time, as you near some high-tension power lines, the pathway will come to an end. Watch for a trail leading up to a nicely designed metal gate inset with river rocks. Walk through this gate and turn right. You're back on Fletcher, walking across the Fletcher Drive Bridge, where a metal plaque will tell you that the bridge was constructed and opened in 1927.

Once across the bridge, continue under the freeway to find your starting point on the corner of Fletcher and Riverside Drive.

Optional Walk Extensions

OPTION #1: Instead of crossing the bridge and heading back toward Riverside, stay on the river walk and use the sloping river bank—watch your step here if it's damp out, and consider avoiding this if it's raining—to cross underneath Fletcher. From there, continue until the river walk crosses under the 5 freeway. From there, you can explore Bowtie Parcel, Taylor Yard, and the back side of Rio De Los Angeles Park. Keep in mind, however, that it will be many miles to the next opportunity to cross back over to the west side of the river.

OPTION #2: Once across Fletcher Bridge, cross Fletcher at Crystal Street and walk through Great Heron Gate into Rattlesnake Park. A short distance down the western side of the river's bikeway, you will see a sign reading "River Access Point," designating the put-in for public boating on the Los Angeles River. If boating is in season, it will say so—a large sign reading "Open for Season" will be spray-painted directly on the concrete bank of the river.

Kayaking on the river only became legal in about 2012, and this part of the river opened for public boating in 2013. The part of the waterway that is legally navigable is only a couple of miles, but it's such a charming little kayak ride, and such a promising glimpse of water use to come, that it's worth a look.

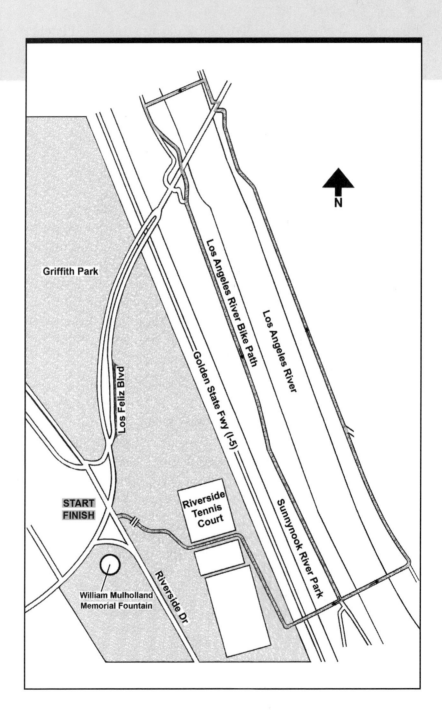

WALK #3

L.A. RIVER WALK NORTH
DISTANCE: **2 miles**
DIFFICULTY: **1**
DURATION: **45 minutes**
DETAILS: **Free parking. Dogs on leash allowed. Wheelchair accessible. Metro buses #96, #180, and #181.**

This section of the Los Angeles River was among the first to receive attention from activists who wanted to turn the waterway back into something other than an ugly concrete channel. The result: one of the city's first new river greenways, and a wonderful place to introduce yourself to the city's watery roots. It's also a good place for a picnic on a hot day.

Begin this walk near the intersection of Riverside Drive and Los Feliz Boulevard, taking advantage of free parking on the street and in the lot that serves the Griffith Riverside tennis courts and soccer field. (Note that this lot is usually crowded on the weekends.)

Before beginning this walk, take in some Los Angeles history at the charming William Mulholland Memorial Fountain in the park on the southeast corner of Riverside and Los Feliz. This fountain has been in this park for decades. On the weekend, it attracts photographers with bands of brides, grooms, and their wedding parties. At night, it's a multi-colored light show, with the sparkling fountain spray transforming under a rainbow of hues.

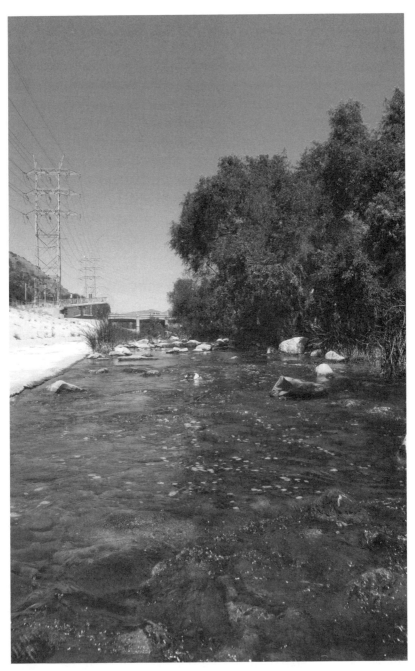

Natural islands have formed in the man-made river.

The watery monument has recently been improved to include a miniature representation of the mighty Los Angeles Aqueduct, the ambitious creation of William Mulholland, the city water engineer who conceived the plan to pipe the precious resource from eastern California's Owens Valley all the way to dry Los Angeles. The resulting construction—223 miles of canals, tunnels, and conduits—is reconstructed here in miniature. Now, at this location, you can "walk" the entire aqueduct in five minutes, and then stand inside an actual piece of the aqueduct pipeline.

To begin your walk, start at the Griffith Riverside tennis facility and soccer field parking lot. Walk toward the tennis reservation booth and take the path just to the left of it, walking between the tennis courts, toward the (increasingly loud) roar of the Golden State Freeway (I-5).

After you've passed the tennis courts, turn right onto a path that parallels the freeway. Walk behind the soccer field, pausing to admire the cleverly designed fake "grass" on the field. Then take the concrete ramp that rises up to the left and carries you above the freeway and over the rushing lanes. On the other side, turn right onto the Los Angeles River Bike Path, taking care not to get run over by cyclists.

Just ahead on the right is one of the city's newer parklets, Sunnynook River Park, which opened in 2013. The area features pathways and benches set amidst a pleasant and botanically accurate display of local flora. All of the plants installed here are native—even the poison oak, which the park designers actually included in their plant palette. (Perhaps one of the informational plaques can explain why the designers were moved to include this particular weed. Maybe it's meant to discourage the homeless people from camping here, as they did before this area was landscaped.)

Once you've admired the park, backtrack a bit to find the narrow Sunnynook Pedestrian Bridge crossing over the river. Cross this bridge, taking a moment to admire the river below. For decades, this was a nasty concrete channel with sludge and crud at its bottom. It was a final resting place for plastic bags, shopping carts, and other urban detritus. A tree would some-times find root here. But then earth movers and other heavy equipment would come in and dredge the channel clean.

Then a group of locals, who eventually called themselves Friends of the L.A. River, began organizing clean-up days and lobbying the city to allow the river to return to its natural state. That's why, as you cross the river now, you see trees and bush-es and the birds that live in them—herons, egrets, ducks, geese, stilts, and other fowl bobbing and darting about. (Underwater, you could find carp, catfish, tilapia, and even trout, I am told.)

Once across the river, turn left and begin walking north along its bank—with the river on your left. If the weather is very dry and there's no chance of rain, you may walk down the slope to the water's edge and get a closer look at the birds. But beware: the mossy parts are very, very slippery, and you must never leave the high bank if it's raining or looks likely to rain. In a heavy rainstorm, this channel will swell to nearly the top of the bank, and people do get swept away from time to time.

Walking north, in time you will see some benches and dis-plays of yoga positions in the shade to your right. The handi-work of the Friends of the L.A. River, this is a good place to have a picnic.

Soon you will find yourself running out of walkway. Step through the gate on your right that leads onto a wide, green field shaded by huge sycamore trees, and walk to Los Feliz Boulevard. (If you come to the end of the fence and find a locked gate, go back twenty-five feet and walk left until you find the opening in the fence.)

Walk straight ahead across a grassy patch, then turn right when you hit the sidewalk. Walk a half block to the traffic light, then cross Los Feliz Boulevard and turn left. As you pass the Los Feliz Café—known to locals as "Eats," because of the big sign—turn into the parking lot. Keep the tiny 9-hole Los Feliz Golf Course on your right, and head for the back of the parking lot. Find a break in the fence, and a paved ramp headed for the river.

Turn right, and enjoy a long flat walk here on the riverbank.

Though it's somewhat obscured by a flood wall, the water below is teeming with life—birds, fish, and in some places, humans and their encampments. On the right, the golf course will end, and a series of horse barns will begin. Many of the city's equestrians stable their horses here.

Rising before you is the L.A. River's newest bridge, a gleaming steel and wood-beam structure, opened in early 2020. Use this to cross to the western side of the water, then turn left and continue your river walk as you go south.

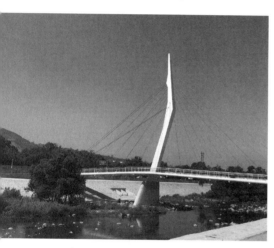

A rarity in Los Angeles, this bridge accommodates pedestrians on one side and equestrians on the other as they cross the L.A. River.

In time you will approach Los Feliz Boulevard again, and a bicycle/pedestrian intersection. Bear left, and walk up a ramp that will keep you on the bike path but carry you up and over Los Feliz. Descend, staying mindful of the cyclists, and continue south.

In this section of the riverbank (known as the Glendale Narrows), you can cut out some of the freeway noise and get closer to the birds by descending the concrete bank to the flank of the river itself—but again, only if the weather is very dry.

As you walk along, enjoy the birds that occupy the small islands in the stream. When you get close to Sunnynook River Park and the narrow pedestrian bridge you used to cross the river a while ago, look right for the pedestrian bridge leading over the freeway. Use this to find your way back to the soccer field and the tennis court reservation booth. Then you'll see the parking lot, and your starting point.

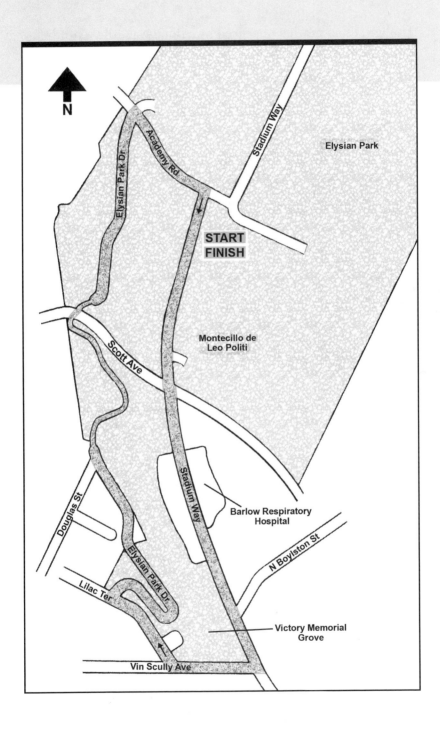

WALK #4

ELYSIAN PARK & BARLOW HOSPITAL
DISTANCE: **2.3 miles**
DIFFICULTY: **2**
DURATION: **1 hour**
DETAILS: **Ample free street parking.
Dogs on leash allowed.
Metro buses #2, #4, #302,
and #704. Avoid this walk on
Dodger game days.**

This is a good leg-stretch that offers some great open spaces near downtown L.A. and some interesting L.A. history from the early 1900s. For a longer hike, this walk pairs up nicely with the Elysian Park & Grace E. Simons Lodge Walk (see Walk #6), which begins nearby.

Begin this walk in Elysian Park, near the intersection of Academy Road and Stadium Way, taking advantage of the ample street parking on Stadium or the parking lot just north of Academy.

Start walking south (downhill) on Stadium, along an avenue with stately date palms lining both sides of the wide street. On the west side, you'll find picnic tables, drinking fountains, play structures, public restrooms, and other amenities. Along the east side, you'll find more picnic tables and a drinking fountain or two.

If you're on the east side, you'll notice a sign for "Montecillo de Leo Politi." This is not a miniature Jeffersonian Monticello (note the different spelling), but a small park-inside-a-park

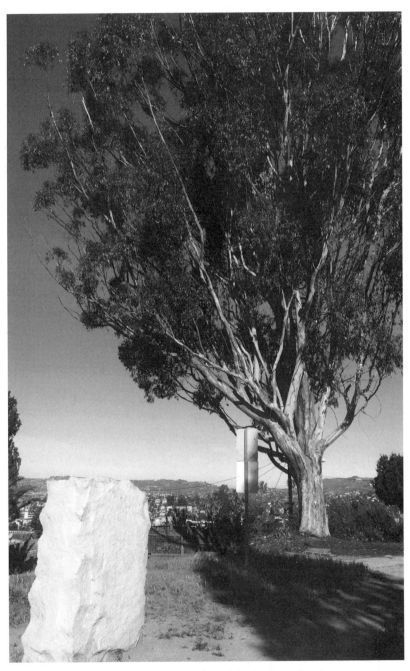

A plinth erected by the Daughters of the American Revolution
in the Victory Memorial Garden.

dedicated to local nature lover and children's book writer Leo Politi, who was also author of *Tales of the Los Angeles Parks*. This mini-park is open between dawn and 3 PM, according to the city. If you wish, explore this area before continuing your walk.

Make your way along the gradual downward slope of Stadium Way, across Scott Avenue, and onto the grounds of the Barlow Respiratory Hospital. Formerly the Barlow Sanitarium, this oasis for tuberculosis patients was founded in 1902 by Walter Jarvis Barlow, who had come west looking for a cure for his own respiratory ailments. He purchased a twenty-five-acre parcel of land from wealthy L.A. landowner J. B. Lankershim for $7,300, and began construction. A man of prodigious energies, Barlow would go on to found the Los Angeles Philharmonic Orchestra and act as dean of the newly formed UCLA School of Medicine.

Much remains of the historic medical campus, despite an ongoing campaign by developers to turn this swath of Elysian Park into a massive condo project. (An equally fierce ongoing campaign by those opposed to the development has kept it from starting for more than a decade.) An inscription on a big chunk of granite near the hospital entrance explains that Barlow founded the hospital and gave it all he had, including the "endless wine of sympathy."

Other metal plaques affixed to buildings state that the original architects were B. B. Bixby and Edward L. Mayberry, whose 1902 work is now afforded Historic-Cultural Monument status, and that the Daughters of the American Revolution dedicated at least two outbuildings to the American Red Cross for "Soldiers and Sailors" just after the first World War.

The hospital, though diminished in importance, is still in use, and still occupied by patients. Several campus buildings are used for teaching and administration. But most of the charming Craftsman bungalows on the west side of the street are boarded up.

Continue along Stadium past this charming time capsule and past North Boylston Street, and climb a short hill to reach

Vin Scully Avenue.

For an amusing side trip, turn left at the corner, into Dodger Stadium's Sunset Gate. A guard will ask to see your identification, then give you a little sticker that will allow you to walk across the vast parking lot and visit the stadium gift shop—and take a look at the empty baseball field.

Otherwise, turn right onto Vin Scully Avenue, climb, climb a little more, and then turn right again onto Lilac Terrace.

Up ahead, you'll see a sign for Victory Memorial Grove. That's your destination. Follow Lilac Terrace up a slight rise, staying on the uphill half of this divided road, past some pleasant shingled bungalows in need of some TLC. At the top of the hill, turn right into the park just before you reach a wide, gated driveway. You'll find yourself on a narrow, partially paved walkway.

Follow this path as it winds across the lower section of the Victory Memorial Grove, under some deodara, oak, and bay laurel shade, and enjoy the views of downtown L.A. Stay with the path as it switchbacks up and left, turning the view into a Dodger Stadium vista. Cross a paved road, climb a short brick staircase, and follow the narrow path as it climbs a short rise. At the plateau, on a hillside dotted with pines and eucalyptus, you will find bigger views of Dodger Stadium and the Barlow Hospital compound.

Near the path, you will encounter a large stone plinth. The inset metal plaque states that it was placed here in 1921 by, again, those Daughters of the American Revolution, to commemorate the family members of their society who lost their lives in World War I.

Return to the path and continue as it drops down a couple of crumbling steps onto the shady residential end of Elysian Park Drive. Walk on, across the intersection with Douglas Street, keeping to the right past a wide white gate to veer right and downhill to another section of Elysian Park Drive.

Up and to the left is a tree-pocked hillside where, if you like, you can get an interesting backside view of Saint Andrew's Ukrainian Orthodox Church, whose golden domes are visible from Sunset Boulevard as it winds through Echo Park.

Otherwise, remain on the paved road as it winds downhill. When you meet Scott Avenue, cross the street, walk around another wide gate, and continue along this closed section of Elysian Park Drive.

Below you are the grassy slopes of Elysian Park. Above are hillsides covered in oak and pepper trees. Straight ahead, along the paved road, you will ultimately meet Academy Road once more. Turn right and head downhill, past another gallery of old date palms and new plantings of their baby siblings.

At the bottom of the hill, you will meet Stadium Way once again, and find yourself back at your starting point.

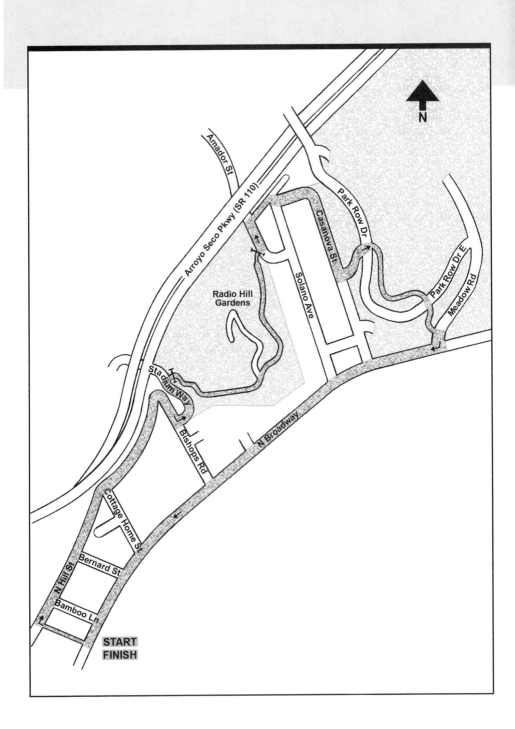

Amador St

Arroyo Seco Pkwy (SR 110)

Park Row Dr

Casanova St

Park Row Dr E

Meadow Rd

Radio Hill
Gardens

Solano Ave

N

Stadium Way

Bishops Rd

N Broadway

Cottage Home St

N Hill St

Bernard St

Bamboo Ln

**START
FINISH**

WALK #5

ELYSIAN PARK & RADIO HILL
DISTANCE: **3.5 miles**
DURATION: **1 hour 30 minutes**
DIFFICULTY: **3**
DETAILS: **Free and metered street parking. Dogs on leash allowed. Metro buses #28, #45, and #83.**

Steps away from busy Chinatown is a walk into a quiet section of wooded hillside, along a trail that rises to fantastic views of downtown and East Los Angeles. A bonus? Good Chinese food before or after the walk.

Begin this walk on North Broadway, near Bamboo Lane, at the historic "Old Chinatown" gate. (Note: This name is slightly bogus. The "old" Chinatown was actually near where Union Station is today, and was razed to make way for the construction of the train station. This Chinatown was built in 1938, in part using Hollywood movie sets donated by Cecil B. DeMille.)

Walk through the "Chinese" plaza, which is part hokey tourist attraction and part working community, filled with shops selling trinkets and apothecaries selling Chinese herbs and medicines.

Emerge on the other side, onto Hill Street, and take a right. Walk about three blocks, past Bamboo Lane and Bernard Street. When it looks like Hill is going to merge with the freeway, veer right to reach the intersection of Cottage Home Street. Jog slightly left, and follow the street as it parallels the freeway and turns into Bishops Road.

On the right, you'll see a large piece of real estate that houses Saint Bridget's Catholic Church and Cathedral High School, a Christian Brothers preparatory school for underprivileged boys that has been operating since 1925. This is the home of the Cathedral Phantoms, so called because the property on which the school was built was once the old Calvary Cemetery. Just out of sight, behind the school buildings, is the school's football field, marked "Cathedral" on one end and "Phantoms" on the other. Their mascot is a skeleton, wrapped in a shroud.

Follow Bishops Road as it rises and winds to the right. Turn left onto Stadium Way, and follow the street up and around a curve. (Again, it will look like you're heading onto the freeway. Don't worry, you aren't.) As the road rises, hook back to the right onto a wide, paved road that is closed to car traffic, and walk past a white security gate. Begin following this flat section of the road as it winds around the hillside to the left.

Already you will see some interesting views: the L.A.

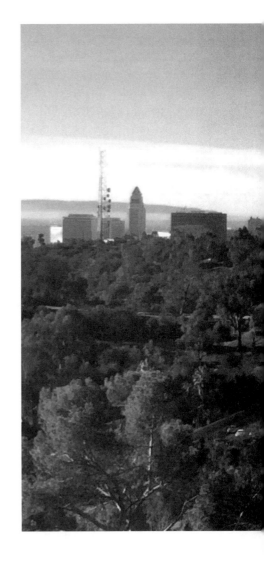

A view of East Los Angeles and the downtown skyline from the top of the hill.

skyline, Union Station, the above-ground stretch of the Gold Line subway, and Los Angeles State Historic Park (nicknamed "The Cornfield" in the 1870s, it is said, after seeds spilling from passing trains sprouted on the site).

As you continue around the hillside, you'll find that the road divides into two paths. For a quick look at the view, take the left-hand road and climb to the technical peak of Radio Hill,

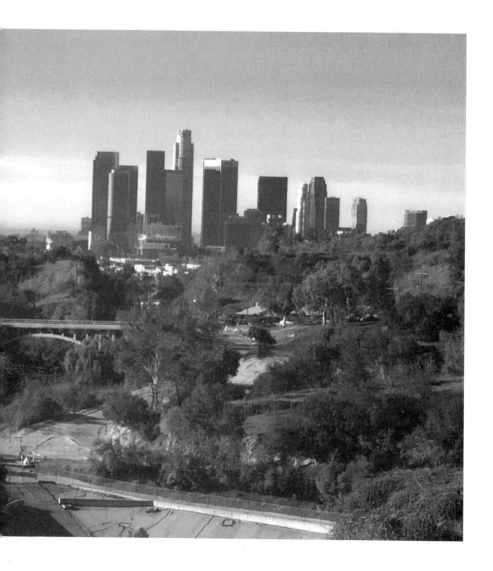

which is home to a large radio tower. After surveying the view, walk back down to the fork and take the other road to continue around the hill.

This piece of paved road will culminate at another low, white security gate. Pass this and cross Amador Street, walking past another white security gate as the paved road, still closed to cars, continues on the other side. This very short stretch will end in the shadow of the freeway. Walk straight on for half a block to meet Solano Avenue.

Veer right on Solano, turning away from the freeway, then turn left at once onto Casanova Street. Walk a short, steep block uphill, then follow the street as it bends to the right and descends. Enter the park on your left at the first opportunity, through a gate onto a series of terraced lawns. Rise from one lawn to the next using the old staircases, or follow the stretch of roadway. Climb past the gate at the top of the hill, and turn right onto Park Row Drive.

Here you will find another terrace of sorts, where the road splits into two. Above this is a narrow dirt trail. Follow it to the right as it parallels the roadway, and walk toward a wide open, sloping lawn.

This is a good picnic spot or, again, a good place to simply enjoy the view. All of downtown L.A., from the skyscrapers on your right to East Los Angeles on your left, is laid out here. It's a good place to sit and speculate, throw a ball for your dog, fly a kite, or . . . continue walking.

The trail will wind around the side of the hill. Follow the lawn downhill, to meet Park Row Drive again. Turn left. Find a narrow path heading downhill on the right, through a series of landscaped terraces. In time, they will drop you onto Meadow Road. Turn right, heading downhill. When you reach North Broadway, turn right again, and head toward downtown.

As you turn, notice the historic marker on your right, indicating this spot as the start of the Portola Trail. This is the beginning of Walk #7 (Elysian Park's Freeway Flyer) in this book, and also an important historical location. The marker indicates the trail used by Don Gaspar de Portola, a Spanish explorer, soldier, and, late in his life, governor of Baja and Alta California. In 1769, he and a small army, sent by the Spanish crown to expel the Jesuits from the missions of California, camped on the banks of what is now the Los Angeles River. Traveling with the Franciscan missionaries Father Juan Crespi and Father Junipero Serra (the latter following in a separate group), Portola marched west from here to the coast, eventually walking all the way to Monterey.

This stretch of noisy roadway is not as nice as the trail to Radio Hill, but it does have its charms. Shortly, on your right, you will see the temple of the Xuan Wu San Buddhist Association. Soon after, you will pass Casa Italiana and Saint Peter's Italian Catholic Church. The former offers dinner and opera shows; the latter hosts regular Sunday Mass. Both serve as a reminder—as did Little Joe's Italian Restaurant, now demolished but formerly located down Broadway a bit—of a time when this neighborhood was more Italian than Chinese.

Continue down the road, passing Cottage Home Street and Bernard Street. If you're curious about the Chinese community here, turn right onto Bernard, where you will find the Chinese Historical Society of Southern California on your right. Otherwise, walk on for another block to the Old Chinatown gates, and find your starting point.

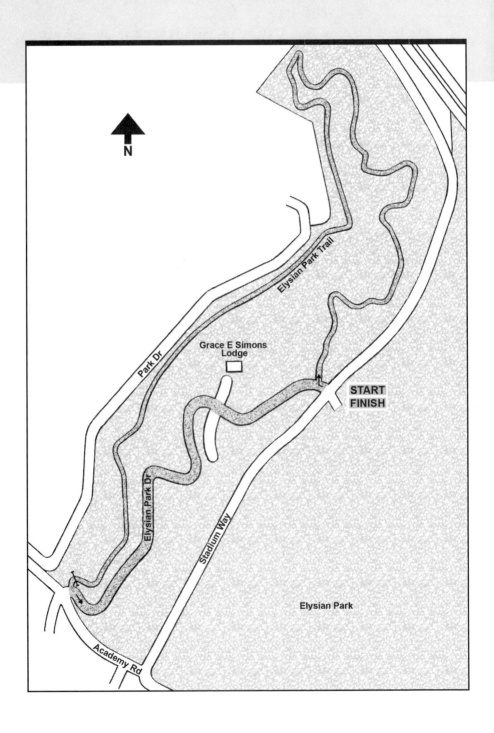

WALK #6

ELYSIAN PARK & GRACE E. SIMONS LODGE
DISTANCE: **2.5 miles**
DURATION: **1 hour**
DIFFICULTY: **3**
DETAILS: **Ample free parking.**
Dogs on leash allowed.
Metro buses #2 and #302.

Here's a hearty city hike that makes a big circle around the heart of Elysian Park. It features good birding, fantastic downtown and northern views, and can be done without crossing any of the park's paved roadways.

Begin this walk in the shadow of Dodger Stadium, on Stadium Way near the corner of Elysian Park Drive.

Follow the signs for Grace E. Simons Lodge, a community center named after Echo Park's most storied activist. It was Ms. Simons—a newspaper reporter who in 1939 began working for one of the city's African-American newspapers—who spearheaded the Citizens Committee to Save Elysian Park. This organization's noisy protest prevented the 1960s development of a convention center in the middle of the park and, later, a football stadium.

Near the corner of Elysian Park Drive and Stadium Way, find a wide trail going up the grassy slope. Walk up this gentle grade, passing under a grove of eucalyptus trees, gaining a little altitude as you go.

This is Elysian Park Trail, one of many named trails in the

550-acre park. It will parallel Stadium Way, and lift you slowly along the hillside. Stay to the right as smaller trails peel away to the left, remaining on the wide dirt path.

As you gain altitude, you will get a better sense of the size of the park. You will also begin to get some good views of the San Gabriel Mountains and the communities north of downtown L.A. You'll get a look at the L.A. River and Taylor Yard, where the city's trains go to sleep at night, as well as Rio de Los Angeles Park, the new park carved out of old Taylor Yard territory. See the swath of greenery on a facing hillside, the one with old-looking buildings on it? That's Forest Lawn Memorial Park in Glendale.

In time, the wide trail will hit a hairpin turn and curve back to the left, climbing more sharply. Follow this up and up, past some houses on the right, and perhaps the smell of horses. People have lived here so long, believe it or not, that one or two of the properties have grandfathered in the right to maintain stables.

After passing a big water tank on the right, you'll reach the crest of the hill. Pause at the charming little spot, known as the Marian Harlow Memorial Garden, where you'll find a bench, a drinking fountain, a dog dish or two, and a "lost and found" for dropped keys, cell phones, etc. Admire the views from here. This is the high point (literally) of the walk. It's all downhill from here.

When you're done, return to the wide Elysian Park Trail and bear left. Begin following the trail as it winds downhill.

The shade is deeper here, and you'll find a thicker mixture of the classic Southern California combo of eucalyptus, pine, oak, and so on. Enjoy the passing parade of red-tailed hawks, great horned owls, woodpeckers, crows, ravens, scrub jays, and California quail.

The trail will parallel the palm-lined Park Drive, uphill and on the right, a great free seat for the fireworks that accompany summer ball games at Dodger Stadium. As you follow the trail, you will also have a nice overlook of the Grace E. Simons Lodge, with its gardens and flowing fountain. People get married at this location, which also hosts bar mitzvahs and other special events.

Walk on, staying on the main trail as it hugs the hillside and descends. In time, you will come to a wide gate. Walk around the gate, make a hard left where the trail meets Academy Road, and walk past another gate onto a stretch of badly worn asphalt.

This is actually part of Elysian Park Drive, no longer open to car traffic. Walk along this road, noting as you go some of the man-made features of the park—a bocce ball court and a children's play area among them.

You will come across one more gate leading into a parking area, beyond which you'll find picnic tables, barbecue grills, and public restrooms. On your left is Grace E. Simons Lodge. Bear right and continue following Elysian Park Drive as it winds back around to approach Stadium Way. When you hit Stadium Way, you will find yourself back at your starting point.

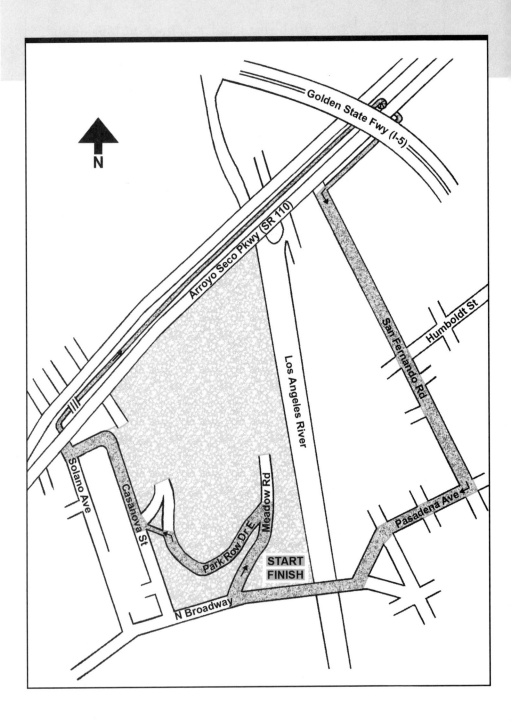

```
┌─────────────────┐
│    WALK #7      │
└─────────────────┘
```

ELYSIAN PARK'S FREEWAY FLYER
DISTANCE: **2.5 miles**
DURATION: **1 hour**
DIFFICULTY: **3**
DETAILS: **Free parking. Dogs on leash allowed. Metro buses #28, #45, and #83.**

The grittiest and most urban of the walks in this collection, this freeway-close stroll is not for the faint of heart. It includes, along with some bucolic greenery and some delightful city views, the roar of the freeway and paths that run through industrial districts adjacent to some homeless encampments. It's perfectly safe, but it's no walk in the park.

Begin this walk at the northeastern entrance to Elysian Park, where North Broadway meets Meadow Road, near where North Broadway crosses the Los Angeles River.

Park on Meadow Road, and return to the corner of North Broadway. There you will find a bronze plaque commemorating the start of the Spanish conquest of Southern California—the spot where the explorer Don Gaspar de Portola, in the company of soldiers and missionaries, camped by the river in 1769 before beginning his march of conquest to Monterey.

Walk uphill on Meadow Road until you meet the first turning. Take a hairpin left onto Park Row Drive East and continue walking uphill on a wide asphalt road, being mindful of the occasional car that might pass.

On your left, you will see some good-looking mature trees and clumps of bougainvillea. On your right is a high, grassy lawn dotted with eucalyptus and oak trees. Straight ahead are the tower atop Radio Hill—part of Walk #5 in this book—and a fine northeasterly version of the downtown Los Angeles skyline.

As the road flattens, look for a low stone drinking fountain on the left, with a narrow asphalt path heading downhill. Take this path a short distance, to the corner of Park Row Drive and Casanova Street, and walk uphill on Casanova. Take note of the charming, fenced-off park on the right, where gnarled old eucalyptus trees decorate a terraced garden, and of the elderly Craftsman and Victorian homes across the canyon—a remnant of a time when Solano Avenue was considered a good address.

Casanova will climb, turn left, and head downhill. Follow along as it does so, then turn right onto Solano Avenue. It will look like you're heading onto a freeway on-ramp. Have no fear. Just stay on the sidewalk, going past the gates of the neighborhood community garden.

Follow the sidewalk as it bends right and leads to steps going down into one of the city's few remaining pedestrian "subway" tunnels, a footpath running under the freeway that helps school kids get from one side of Solano Canyon to the other. This is a relatively clean and well-lit place, running for 100 feet underground.

On the other side, emerge up a flight of stairs and make a hairpin right turn. Go through a gate and up a series of staircases, walking parallel to the northbound freeway (the lanes you've just walked under). Continue to the top of the stairs, where you will meet the southbound freeway lanes and, through a swing gate, one of Los Angeles's weirdest public walkways.

Below you is the original Arroyo Seco Parkway (SR 110), the first freeway in the Western United States. There used to be just one road running from Pasadena into downtown. It was a broadened expansion of the old Figueroa Street that cut through the hills via four tunnels built in the 1930s. Then, in the 1940s, when traffic outgrew the Parkway's original four lanes, the

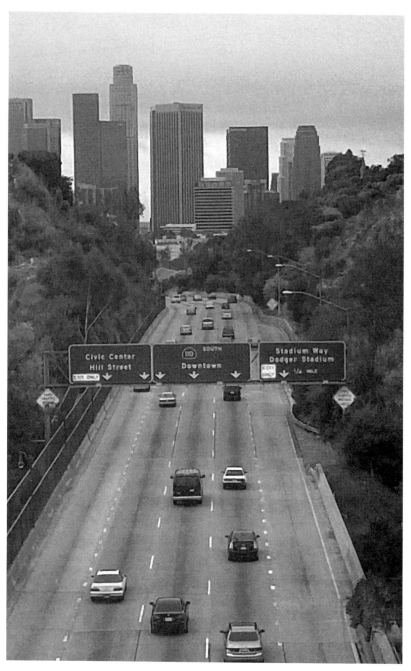

A view of downtown L.A. from above the freeway.

roadway was doubled to include what are now the southbound lanes—the lanes uphill to your left.

Because this new construction eliminated the pedestrian sidewalks that had run alongside Figueroa, a new sidewalk was built, running parallel to the southbound freeway lanes—in effect, halfway between the two sides of the roaring expressway.

Turn right into this narrow, fenced-off walkway, and begin walking north toward the southbound traffic. (For future walks, or to extend this one, note that this walkway runs all the way into Chinatown if you head south.) On your right side, you will see concrete walls overgrown with Boston ivy. Above you are elegant bridges and period lamp posts. And to your left, seemingly inches away, are automobiles moving at sixty miles per hour—unless it's rush hour, when they're barely moving at all.

The walkway will pass beside some well-established homeless encampments down the slopes to the right (behind a chain-link fence). As you go, it will also offer increasingly broad views of the mountains above Pasadena and Altadena. Eventually it will emerge and present even broader views of the Los Angeles River, the massive County Hospital in East Los Angeles, and the train lines and Gold Line subway line running up from downtown.

The sidewalk will end at a circular staircase above the complex merging of the Arroyo Seco Parkway and the Golden State Freeway (I-5). Take the staircase the equivalent of several floors down to an intersection of several pathways. Walk straight on from here, beside what is now the fast lane of the northbound freeway.

As you walk along, you will get a perhaps too-close look at the ironwork that supports the southbound freeway lanes, as well as an uglier stretch of the concrete-lined L.A. River.

Walk on. The sidewalk will end again in another hairpin turn, this time to the left. Drop down a (sometimes very dirty) set of stairs, and at the bottom turn left onto San Fernando Road.

This will lead you past a freeway onramp and, a few blocks on, underneath the Gold Line tracks as they head toward the Lincoln Heights/Cypress Park Station. This section of San Fernando, which is also part of historic Route 99—the state's main north–south highway before the I-5 was built—isn't particularly beautiful. But it will treat you to views of the vehicle storage yards for the Department of Sanitation, the Fire Department, and the Department of Transportation, all on your right.

On your left, you'll find a couple of thrift store options: Goodwill Industries, with its period "Not Charity But A Chance" sign, and, to the left up Humboldt Street, a Saint Vincent de Paul Society outlet. You'll also have several chances to fill your medical marijuana prescription.

Turn right from San Fernando onto Pasadena Avenue. Walk a few blocks, past the massive Young Nak Presbyterian Church compound across the street to your left, until Pasadena meets North Broadway. Turn right, pass the gates of the city, and cross the elegant Buena Vista Street Viaduct, a 1909 bridge over the L.A. River.

Here you'll find lovely views of the downtown skyline and Los Angeles State Historic Park, also known as "The Cornfield" (so nicknamed in the 1870s, the story goes, after seeds spilling from passing trains sprouted on the site).

On the other side of the bridge, near the Portola Trail marker, turn right onto Meadow Street. You are back at your starting point.

PART TWO

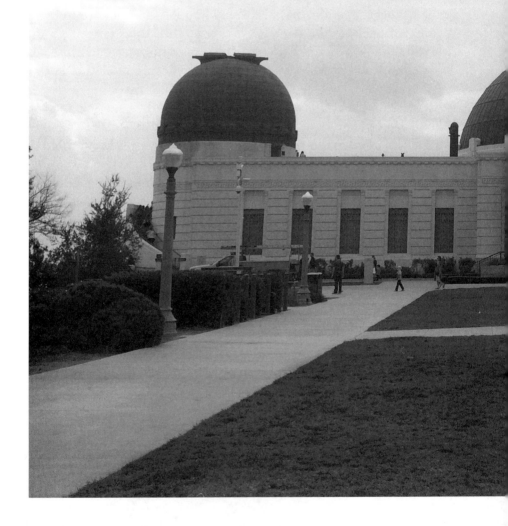

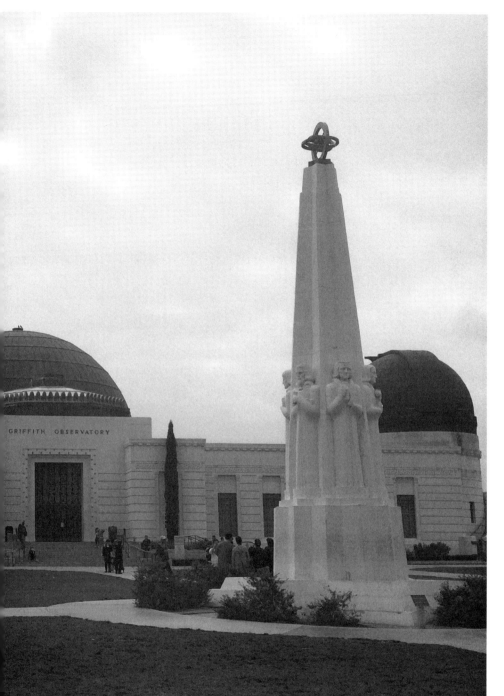

GRIFFITH PARK

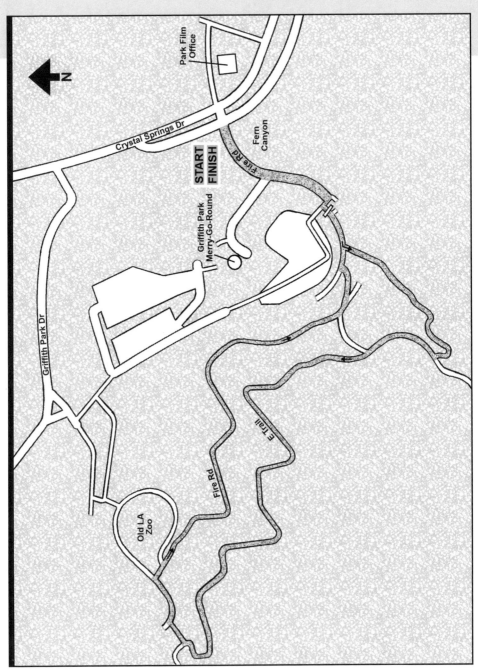

Overleaf: The Observatory, inside Griffith Park.

WALK #8

THE OLD ZOO
DISTANCE: **2.5 miles**
DIFFICULTY: **2**
DURATION: **1 hour**
DETAILS: **Free parking. Dogs on leash allowed. Metro bus #96.**

On this walk, a series of wide, easy trails through the city's largest park leads to the ruins of the city's original zoo, and the site of some unusual outdoor performances.

Near the center of Griffith Park, off Crystal Springs Drive, take the short spur road that leads to the parking lot for the park's famed merry-go-round.

Before you set out on your walk, take a minute to admire this fine old contraption, built in 1926 and operating at this location since 1937. It's the real deal, fitted with sixty-eight leaping horses and a band organ capable of playing over 1,500 different marches and songs. The merry-go-round is open on weekends all year round, and weekdays during the summer.

Leave the merry-go-round parking lot the same way you came in, but turn uphill as you do and walk about fifty feet, past the white barricade. Look for a flat trail on your left leading up into a narrow canyon. (There are several paths here. The wrong ones either climb quite quickly or are quite wide. The right one has a deep drainage culvert near its beginning.)

Pass the culvert and walk into a shaded bower, with a few wooden steps gradually giving you a bit of elevation. In a short time, you will come to the Fern Canyon Trail Amphitheater.

Climb a set of wooden stairs out of this, and turn right onto a wide dirt road named East Trail.

The road will descend and then bend left with the contour of the hillside before climbing a bit. As it does, it will parallel the paved road above the merry-go-round and provide views of lower Griffith Park (including the golf courses you may have circumnavigated on Walk #9), the city of Glendale, and, in the distance, the green space that is Forest Lawn Memorial Park.

In time, after about half a mile, the wide trail will make a sharp bend to the right. In the elbow of this bend, find a narrow trail dropping straight down a dry creek bed, shaded by sycamore, oak, and eucalyptus trees. Walk this trail until it hits a stretch of paved road, then turn right.

The lawns before you are part of the Crystal Springs Picnic Area. The sloping section farther along has been host to Shakespeare in the Park performances, as well as the "Symphony in the Glen" outdoor concerts once given by members of the Los Angeles Philharmonic.

Over to the right is something much stranger: the old Los Angeles Zoo.

The zoo has its roots, as so much of the city does, in Hollywood. In the early silent movie days, a filmmaker named William Selig was using so many wild animals in his films that he decided to put them on display on a piece of his property (near what is now Lincoln Park) and charge people to come see them. Slight remnants of this fantastic tourist attraction, including a street named Selig Place, remain in the current park, off North Mission Road, near the Plaza De La Raza.

In 1915, Selig got out of the zoo business and donated his animals to the city. With that, the Los Angeles Zoo opened in its original location in the section of Griffith Park where you are now standing. The property had already been home to an ostrich park owned by Colonel Griffith J. Griffith, the mining magnate who gave the city the land for the park that bears his name. The city operated the zoo in this location until 1956, when it moved to its current, much larger facility—partly in response to a series of articles criticizing the small, inhumane animal enclosures at the original location.

Those small, inhumane enclosures remain here for the public to see.

Walk along the edge of the property's wide lawn to explore the cages and pens where gorillas and elephants once resided. It's not unusual to see an entire family (of humans) picnicking in one of the original animal houses.

When you've had enough of that, walk back uphill to the uppermost animal enclosure and look for a narrow paved path running to the left, behind the animal cages. This will climb up above the cages, revealing how the animal handlers entered the enclosures to feed and water the beasts.

Soon the path will meet a wider, unpaved trail. Walk along this trail, which parallels the hillside-hugging trail you were on a half-hour ago. It will meander back to the merry-go-round parking lot and return you to your starting point.

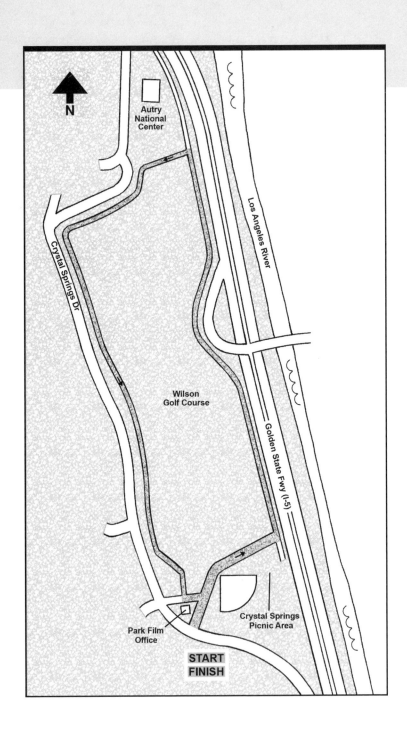

WALK #9

THE GOLF COURSE LOOP
  DISTANCE: **2.5 miles**
  DIFFICULTY: **1**
  DURATION: **1 hour**
  DETAILS: **Free parking. Dogs on leashes allowed. Wheelchair-accessible. Metro bus #96.**

This flat walk along the edge of one of Griffith Park's biggest open green spaces has all the charm of a round of golf, with none of the expense, frustration, or special equipment. No mashies or niblicks are needed to enjoy this golf course loop. (Note that this walk pairs up nicely with Walk #8, the Old Zoo Walk.)

After entering Griffith Park along Crystal Springs Drive, park near the signs for the Crystal Springs Picnic Area or "Poke Field," the beautifully maintained baseball diamond.

To begin your walk, find the wide equestrian path that runs just in front of the Park Film Office and the small Visitors Center. Begin walking downhill on this wide path, away from Crystal Springs Drive and toward the Golden State Freeway (I-5).

As you approach the freeway, the path will hit a T-intersection. Turn left, and begin walking along the golf course on your left. This is a long, clear alley, overhung by old eucalyptus and oak trees and paralleling the Wilson Golf Course—one of Griffith Park's several eighteen-hole courses. (The others are also named after presidents: Harding and Roosevelt.)

For years I have groused that so much of the city's grassy parkland was reserved for the private use of golfers. There should be pedestrian walkways, I said, either inside or alongside these golf courses, so that non-golfers could enjoy these relatively rare swaths of green acreage.

This trail, it turns out, is one such walkway, and allows walkers to share the beauty of the fairways with the golfers without endangering themselves or being a nuisance to the golfers.

The pathway, which is open to horses but not to bicycles or motorized vehicles, runs right alongside the golf course. The lush green grass, even in times of drought, is a cooling, soothing sight, and attracts wildlife (perhaps especially during times of drought). On a warm August morning you might see coyotes and deer wandering through the shady sections, ignoring the golfers and golf carts.

Notice as you go along that the charming split-rail fence on your left is actually made of sections of concrete that are formed to look like wood. This is a crude version of the "faux-bois" handrails common in other parts of Griffith Park, especially the Fern Dell area (see Walk #10). Also notice the large screens along the path, meant to keep errant golf balls from flying onto the freeway. Don't worry—they'll protect you, too.

Walk on until you reach your first intersection. The path straight ahead continues for quite some distance. If you were in the mood for a really long walk, you could continue all the way past the Los Angeles Zoo to the park's Travel Town Museum, which features fully functioning steam locomotives and other railway relics.

For now, though, turn left at this intersection, keeping the green golf course on your left as you enter another alley of eucalyptus trees. In a few minutes, you'll see more lawn area on your right. This is the front of the Autry National Center, also known as the "Cowboy Museum"—a great institution in its own right, and worth a look on another day.

Stay left again where the path splits, keeping the golf course on your left. When you come to a roadway (which is actually another section of Crystal Springs Drive), head left once more, continuing to keep the golf course on your left.

This is the section of roadway where the park used to host its kitschy but charming Department of Water and Power Light Festival, an annual autumnal display of electric lights depicting the geographical, architectural, and artistic highlights of life in Los Angeles: neon surfers, neon buffalo, neon movie stars, etc. The festival has recently been moved inside the grounds of the zoo, where an updated version of the once-free display of L.A.-themed lights now costs money to see.

Continue along, enjoying the sight of golfers and their golf carts and perhaps catching a glimpse of some wildlife. Off to the right, you may catch sight of the park's famed carousel, an ancient merry-go-round that has been in this location since 1937. There are also a couple of tennis courts across the way. On some weekend days, you may also hear drumming coming from the drum circles that form on the drive up to the carousel.

As you approach the end of the loop, you'll come to an outdoor exercise area, filled with rudimentary equipment for various workouts. Continue to the next bend in the pedestrian path, and stop where it turns left again and begins to head downhill toward the freeway. You have completed the loop, and are back at your starting point.

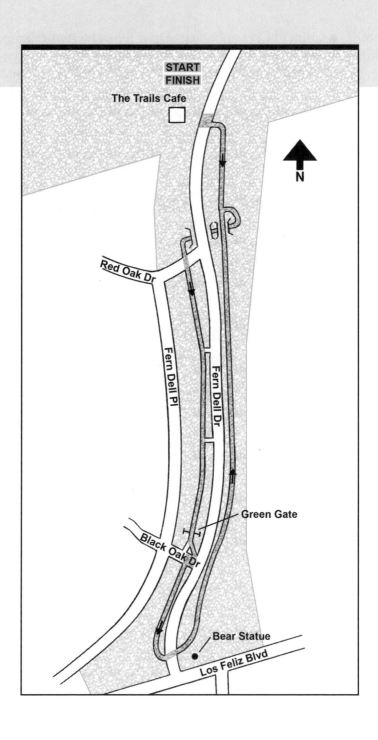

WALK #10

FERN DELL
DISTANCE: **1.25 miles**
DIFFICULTY: **1**
DURATION: **45 minutes**
DETAILS: **Free street parking. Dogs on leash allowed. Wheelchair accessible. Metro buses #207 and #180/#181, and the Hollywood Dash.**

This charming, short walk is the only one I know of in all of Los Angeles that can be done entirely in the shade, even on the sunniest of days. It's perfect on a really hot afternoon, for a quiet stroll along a burbling creek when the rest of the city is baking.

Before beginning this gentle walk, head for the Trails Cafe on Fern Dell Drive—a good place to grab a coffee and a home-baked pastry.

From the cafe, cross Fern Dell Drive into the deeply shaded park area. Here you will find play structures, picnic tables, barbecue pits, public restrooms, and drinking fountains. You will also find a paved path leading into the famed Fern Dell Grotto. Follow this path downhill as it descends gradually into deeper shade.

This canyon was home to Tongva and Gabrielino natives for centuries. At the early part of the twentieth century, though, it was part of the land deeded to the city by Colonel Griffith J.

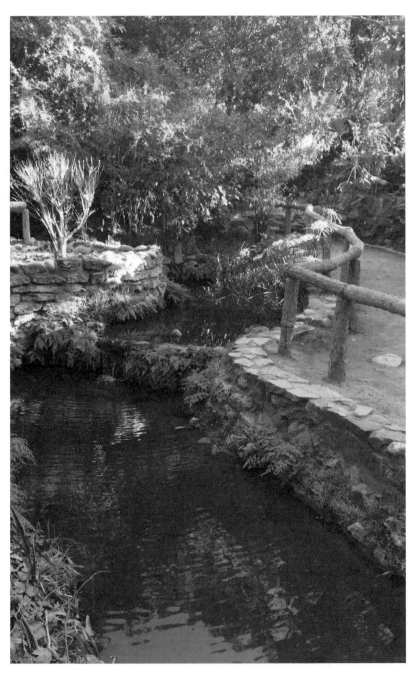

A cool, shady stretch of the Fern Dell trail, lined with "faux-bois" handrails.

Griffith. Starting in about 1914, this little stretch began to be carved into the fabricated natural spot that it is today. Throughout the 1920s and into the Depression, the grotto's pools were dug, its trails were cut, and its plants were imported.

A significant amount of the work was done by Civilian Conservation Corps workers housed in the park, who used National Park Service texts to guide their construction. It is to them that we owe the "faux-bois" handrails—formed concrete, made to look like wood—and terraced pool gardens that you encounter as you walk downhill through this strange, lush, fern-lined canyon, shaded by sycamore, oak, and even redwood trees towering above.

The path will wander along, dropping below grade and crossing underneath Fern Dell Drive. Here and there you will find benches near the pools, in which you can sometimes see small fish playing. (In its heyday, Fern Dell was fed by quite a lively stream. You can see remnants of this farther up the canyon, above your starting point, where even now a dry, river rock-lined stream bed waits for the water to return.)

In time, the path will pass though a set of green gates onto the sidewalk running along Fern Dell Drive. To make a loop, cross Fern Dell—taking note of the small standing bear cub statue on the lawn, a tribute from Los Angeles's sister city, Berlin—and find a wide path running along the hillside to the east of the dell itself. This will lead you back up the canyon, along a series of pleasant spots for picnicking or lounging. It will also lead to a major trail heading off to the right that will ultimately deliver you to the Griffith Park Observatory—if you're in the mood for a much bigger walk (see Walk #11).

For now, turn around and retrace your steps on the trail, soaking up more of the ferny shade as you climb the canyon back to Trails Cafe and your starting point.

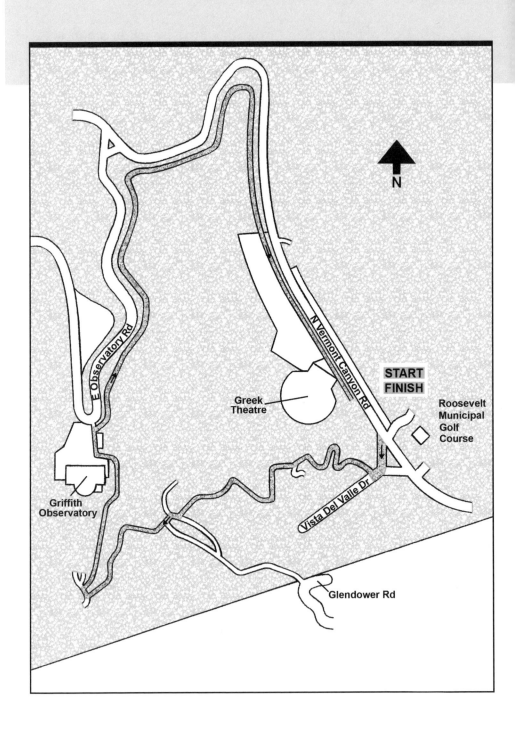

WALK #11

THE OBSERVATORY LOOP
DISTANCE: **1.9 miles**
DIFFICULTY: **4**
DURATION: **1 hour**
DETAILS: **Free street parking.**
Dogs on leash allowed.
Metro buses #180 and #181.

This is a short, steep route from Vermont Canyon to the Observatory and back, using a combination of trails and park roads. It's a great way to see the iconic Observatory building, enjoy its deep-space shows and exhibits, and take in the massive city views from its decks—without having to wait for the shuttle or struggle to find parking. But it's a steep hike, no doubt. Wear good shoes and bring water.

Begin your walk by driving or walking up into Los Feliz's Vermont Canyon, north of Los Feliz Boulevard and above where Vermont Avenue and Hillhurst Avenue merge. Park anywhere around the Greek Theatre or the Roosevelt Municipal Golf Course (but not in the golf course lot, where posted signs indicate that your car may be towed away).

Take advantage of the public restrooms and the interesting selection of snacks, sandwiches, and gourmet groceries at Franklin's Cafe and Market.

Cross Vermont Canyon to the west side and head for the little spur road known on different maps as Vista Del Valle Drive or Boy Scout Drive. This road runs a short straight distance due west and up a slight incline. (The Greek Theatre should be on your right as you approach this incline, with a wide grassy field to your left and the golf course at your back.)

A scant few yards in, turn right onto a wide dirt path shaded by sycamores, leaving the roadway. Head up a steep hill, following this wide path as it begins to switch back on itself and quickly gain elevation. Wind along with it, staying on the main wide path as you cross a series of smaller trails going left and right. You will gradually have better and better views of Vermont Canyon and the Los Feliz neighborhood.

In time, the main dirt path will end at a narrow paved roadway. Turn right, and walk uphill for about seventy-five feet. Then turn left onto another wide dirt path. (If you're exploring, going right on the paved road will take you to a water tower high behind the Greek Theatre. Turning left will take you to a gate leading out of the park, onto Glendower Place.)

The path will climb a little more and come to a flat area under some shade trees, where you will probably find other walkers stopping to admire the view and catch their breath before the last big push to the summit. Make a hairpin right turn and begin the final steep climb to the Observatory itself, keeping the imposing white building on your left.

Once you arrive at the front of the Observatory, depending on how much time you have, stop to admire the views and enjoy what the landmark has to offer.

The Observatory was a gift to the city from Griffith J. Griffith, who also donated the original land for the park named in his honor. After seeing the big telescope at Mount Wilson, Griffith had wanted one of his own. So, in 1912, he donated $100,000 for the construction of an observatory, open to the public for free, so that everyone could look into deep space.

Griffith died in 1919, long before the 1930 completion of his bequest, but his legacy lives on and the city honors his wish. The Observatory is open from noon to 10 PM on weekdays (but closed on Mondays) and from 10 AM to 10 PM on weekends. Entrance is free; ticket prices vary for planetarium shows. The site also offers a variety of free walks, talks, and events.

The best views of the city are from the outside decks on the building's south-facing side. You can also get a coffee or a snack at the Wolfgang Puck-operated cafe on the building's west side.

Return to the front of the Observatory, where you'll find a large stone plinth honoring the great historical names of science. (Over to the west side of the property is a shiny bust of actor James Dean, who is not one of the great names of science, but whose performance in the 1955 film *Rebel Without a Cause* includes a dramatic scene acted out at this location.) With the building at your back, follow the sidewalk on the right side as it leaves the parking lot and begins to slope downward.

Stay to the right, walking in the shade of some old pine trees that have somehow survived the drought and all the brush fires that have burned through here over the years, and begin descending. You'll come to an intersection with a landscaped triangle of land in the middle of it. To the left is a tunnel through the mountain that separates the city from the valley. (For the record, it's also the tunnel that separated the city from Toon Town in the movie *Who Framed Roger Rabbit*.)

Turn right at the intersection, and continue walking downhill. If you have time, cross the street at the big right-hand bend in the road and explore the old bird sanctuary, once as lush and green as the park's Fern Dell Grotto (which you can enjoy in Walk #10). Some of the infrastructure remains, as do areas where ponds and streams once flowed, though the exotic birds have long since flown the coop.

Continue moving south, past the long parking lots for the Greek Theatre. At the stop signs marking the next intersection, slow down and look around. Didn't you leave your car around here somewhere? Yes. You're back at your starting point.

PART THREE

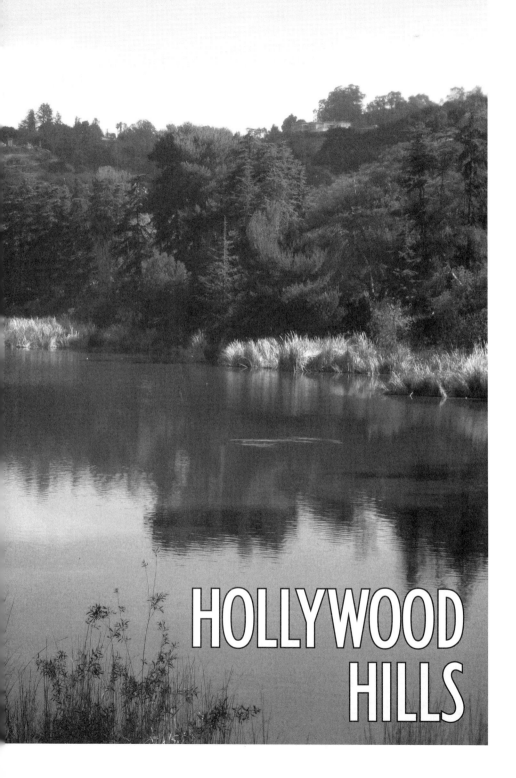

HOLLYWOOD
HILLS

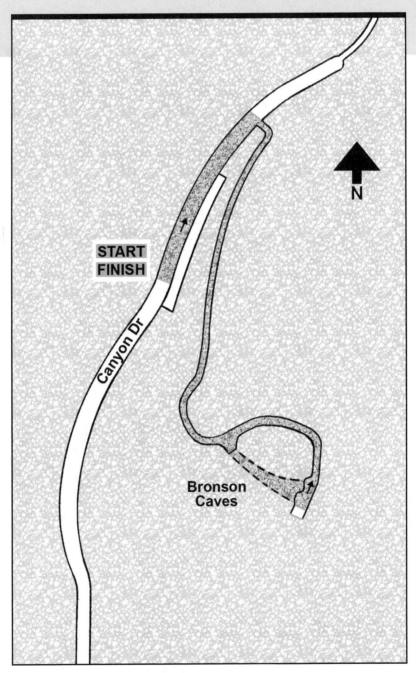

START
FINISH

Canyon Dr

N

Bronson
Caves

Overleaf: A view looking north across the Upper Franklin Canyon Reservoir.

WALK #12

BRONSON CANYON & THE BAT CAVE
DISTANCE: **1 mile**
DURATION: **20 minutes**
DIFFICULTY: **1**
DETAILS: **Free street parking.**
Dogs on leash allowed.
DASH Hollywood.

This is a short but fascinating walk through the Hollywood Hills and some Hollywood history, with a visit to one of the film and TV industry's most famous filming locations—the "Bat Cave" used for the old Batman *TV show and many other onscreen moments.*

Find your way to the top of Canyon Drive, in Hollywood's Bronson Canyon. Park on the street or in the parking lot at the Bronson Canyon entrance to Griffith Park. Then start walking toward the hills.

High above, you will see trails leading toward the Hollywood Sign, and the viewing platform you might have visited in Walk #13. You can also catch glimpses of the Griffith Park Observatory, high up on your right.

Nearer to hand, you will see picnic and play areas on the right as you walk, as well as signs for Camp Hollywoodland, a recreational area for girls, run for decades by the city of Los Angeles.

Walk straight on. Shortly you will come to a right-hand turn. Take this, and walk from paved road onto crusty dirt road. Begin strolling up a slight slope paralleling the road you drove in on.

The road will rise and bend to the left, passing several trails that, for this walk, are to be avoided. Follow the wide dirt road as it broadens and bends left into an open area. Right in front of you is the Bronson Cave—or, as it's more familiarly known, the Bat Cave.

Anyone who grew up in the sixties (I did, too, so you have my sympathy) will recognize this hole in the rock as the secret exit from Batman's home—"stately Wayne Manor," as it was known on the TV show—that was used exclusively as the emergency driveway for the Batmobile. (For the actual "Wayne Manor" filmed for the show, check out Walk 25, in the Arroyo Seco section of Pasadena.) When trouble called, Batman would hop in his ride, throw some secret switch, and *swoosh!* The bushes camouflaging the Bat Cave would be flung aside, and the Batmobile would roar into action.

The cave itself is high and wide, but not very deep. It takes less than a minute to walk through it. In reality, it's hardly big enough to conceal a Batmobile.

This area was originally a quarry, developed for mining. In the early 1900s, the hard rock of the foothills was chipped away by the Union Rock Company to produce some of the stone and gravel used to pave the surrounding streets.

It is said that the Union and subsequent mining companies blasted a hole through the rock to make it easier to transport pieces of it down the hill. Given the layout, however, that's not very logical—not to mention that much of the cave's interior looks natural, rather than manmade.

On the other side of the cave are steep canyon walls, with some goat trails (not recommended at all) leading up to other entrance points in the park. A wide dirt road swings around to the left of the cave and reconnects with the main entrance.

Despite its relatively small size, the Bat Cave has been used countless times in the making of movies and TV shows. Close to the studios, but set in a remote-looking atmosphere, the Bronson Cave (or Caves, since there is a little side cave on the left) has played a starring role in movies as disparate as the 1932 drama *I Am a Fugitive From a Chain Gang*, the 1956 sci-fi classic *Invasion of the Body Snatchers*, and 1991's *Star Trek VI: The Undiscovered Country*.

Many of the movies filmed here have been forgettable, low-budget affairs, such as *Atom Man vs. Superman*, *Earth vs. the Spider*, and *Monster from Green Hell*. But it's also been a working TV set since the earliest days of the medium. Episodes of *Gunsmoke* were filmed here, as were parts of *The Monkees*, *Mission: Impossible*, *Have Gun, Will Travel*, *The Outer Limits*, and Clint Eastwood's *Rawhide*. *Star Trek* used this location in almost every season. So did *Twin Peaks* and *Wonder Woman*.

So, if you feel like you've been here before—you have.

Enjoy the cave. Take a selfie. Check out the views. Check out the wildlife. One morning while walking here I saw a whole family of coyotes, standing rather ominously on the ridge far above the caves.

Then begin your walk back to the main road, going back through the cave or winding your way around the back side of it. Take the wide dirt road back to the paved road, then turn left and make your way downhill and back to your starting point.

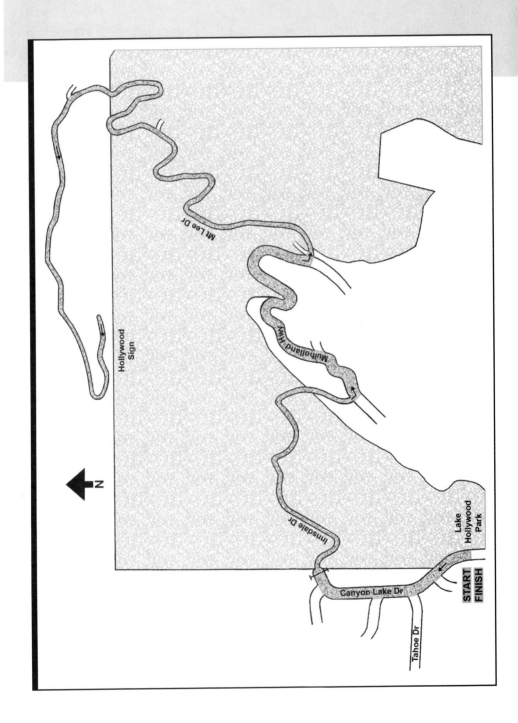

WALK #13

THE HOLLYWOOD SIGN WALK
  DISTANCE: **5 miles**
  DURATION: **2 hours**
  DIFFICULTY: **5**
  DETAILS: **Free street parking.**
  Dogs on leash allowed.
  DASH Beachwood and DASH
  Hollywood.

In recent years, the city has tried to deny automobile access to the areas near the Hollywood Sign by closing streets leading to them, and for a while even built a fence and posted a security guard to discourage pedestrians. But this a great hike that will take you as close to the famous sign as is legally possible. A bonus: Huge views of the city and the San Fernando Valley.

Begin this walk, which is really more of a hike, near Lake Hollywood Park, off Canyon Lake Drive. Park carefully—it's a steep street—then walk downhill. (You might find better parking nearer the bottom of the hill, below the park.) Where you might ordinarily turn left onto Tahoe Drive to get down to the reservoir, walk straight instead as Canyon Lake rises, bends to the right, and stops. Cross the white steel gate and continue walking uphill on Innsdale Drive, on what is now an unpaved stretch of wide roadway.

Suddenly, you'll find yourself in the country, enjoying typical Southern California scenery: dry brush, sloping hillsides, eucalyptus trees, fields of cactus, and increasingly good views of the city below you.

Walk on as Innsdale bends and rises. You will catch glimpses of the Hollywood Sign, which, as history tells us, once read "Hollywoodland" and was erected to advertise a new real estate development in Beachwood Canyon. After the sign became the property of the City of Los Angeles in the forties, the "land" portion of the sign was removed. Since then, the Hollywood Sign has been rebuilt, restored, and maintained as a beloved symbol of the district.

As you walk, you'll notice a couple of narrow trails that spur off from the wide dirt road. Ignore those for now and keep walking, enjoying views of the reservoir known as Lake Hollywood. (For more on that, and a flatter, easier stroll, check out Walk #14.)

In time, Innsdale will narrow and wind between some residences before it hits paved road again. This is Mulholland Highway, a remnant of the scenic roadway that was designed to carry motorists on a ridge above the city, all the way from Hollywood to the sea north of Malibu. Some sections of this highway remain, a few of which are still quite scenic.

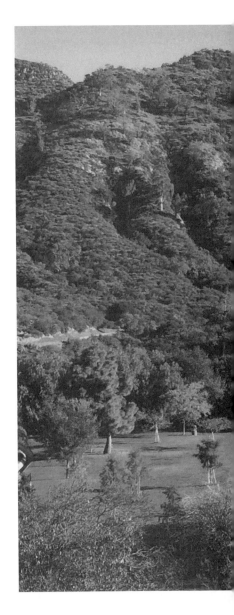

The famous Hollywood Sign, originally an advertisement for a real estate development in the area.

The most well-traveled portions are the stretch between the Hollywood Freeway (U.S. 101) and the San Diego Freeway (I-405), and a section between Topanga Canyon and Kanan Dume Road in the Malibu mountains.

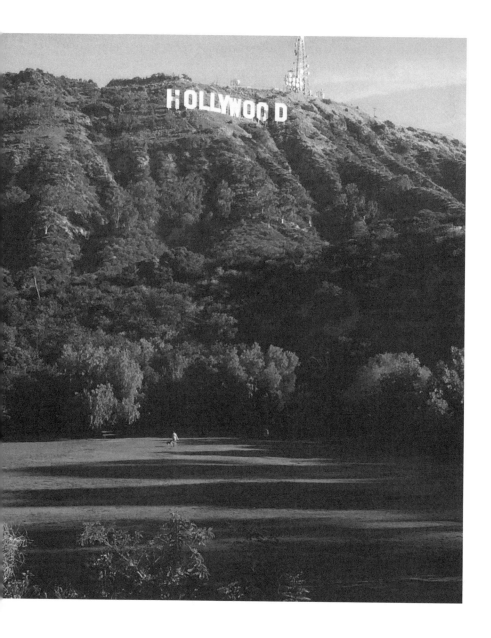

Turn left onto Mulholland, and stay on the uphill side of the street as the road divides. Up and along you will go, snatching better and better views of the Hollywood Sign. You'll probably start to see tourists here, ditching their rented Mustang convertibles by the side of the road to take selfies with the famous sign high above them.

Do not be discouraged if you see signs saying there is no access to the Hollywood Sign, nor by a security guard, if you see one. This area is closed to automobiles, but open for walking. The security guard is looking for troublemakers—not for you.

Walk on. As you go, you'll pass through a pretty residential district with some appealing architectural homes. Soon, it will seem like you're walking right through their front yards. You are, almost. Respect their property and walk straight on, until you come to what looks like the end of the road.

Look to the left. You'll see a pedestrian-only bypass, a little gate. Walk through this, latching it behind you if it's been left open. Then, bearing left, walk down the lower of the two options, a wide, paved section of old roadway. This is Mount Lee Drive.

From here on up, it's a lovely, steady walk, climbing the whole way, but not too steep. You will be graced as you go with changing views and different angles of the big city below.

At the one intersection you will encounter, keep left, staying on Mount Lee Drive. (The road to the right would take you down to either Beachwood Drive and the Bat Cave or all the way into Griffith Park and up to the Observatory.)

Keep climbing. The road will wend and wind, eventually making a big loop as it approaches the summit. Here, your view will shift north, into the valley. Before you are Glendale and Burbank, with the Forest Lawn/Mount Sinai cemetery compound directly downhill. Slightly beyond that are the Disney and Warner Bros. studio lots.

Climb on a bit more. Soon the road will loop back around and deposit you onto a wide platform directly above the Hollywood Sign. Climb yet a bit more and you will reach the very peak. You made it!

This spot is at helicopter level, and some days, you will see police or fire choppers hovering over Hollywood. Other days, you will see private helicopters or, a little higher, private planes, taking tours of the city. Your view is as good as theirs, and you got a workout to boot.

When you've enjoyed the view long enough, head back down the way you came, making sure to bear right at the one intersection. Hook to the right and go back through the pedestrian gate from Mount Lee Drive onto Mulholland.

To make sure you don't miss the turn onto Innsdale, watch for the split in the roadway. Stay to the upper side, on the right. If the roadways merge and become one again, you've gone just a little too far—go back, and turn onto the unpaved Innsdale.

Walk down this road until it meets the paved Canyon Lake Drive again, and follow that as it falls, begins to rise again, and returns you to your starting point.

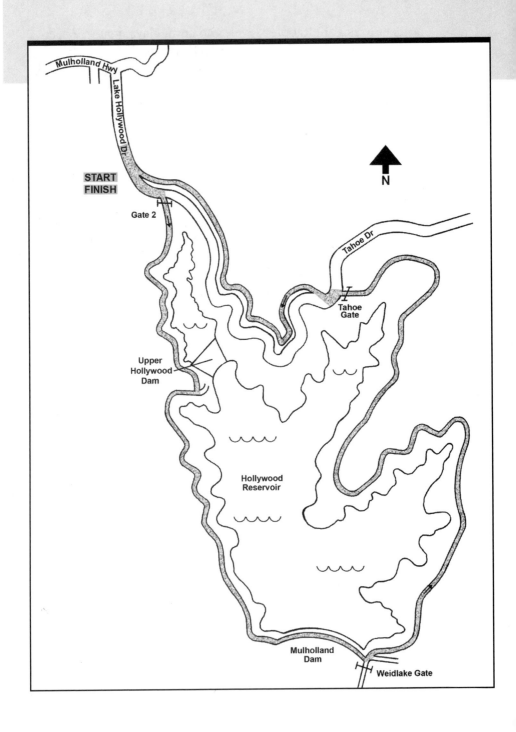

WALK #14

AROUND LAKE HOLLYWOOD
DISTANCE: **3.6 miles**
DURATION: **1 hour 30 minutes**
DIFFICULTY: **1**
DETAILS: **Ample free parking. Open
to bicycles. Closed to dogs.
Wheelchair accessible.**

This flat walk around one of the city's most scenic reservoirs offers a close-up view of the Hollywood Sign and, often, some Griffith Park wildlife.

Begin this walk off Barham Boulevard, at the point where Lake Hollywood Drive descends from Wonder View Drive and meets the northern edge of the reservoir.

Park here and enter the enclosure that surrounds Lake Hollywood. (This is Gate 2, one of three access points to the walkway around the lake.) Begin walking to the right, making a counterclockwise circuit around the water.

This reservoir was the brainchild of William Mulholland, the man who designed the Los Angeles Aqueduct and brought water to the desert. (His story is the basis for the great L.A. noir movie *Chinatown*.) Completed in 1924, the aqueduct was built to supply drinking water to the growing population. After construction of the massive dam, water was flooded into what was then known as Weid Canyon. The Hollywood Reservoir, also known as Lake Hollywood, was born.

The pathway you're on will follow the contour of the lake,

which, unfortunately, is separated from walkers by a chain-link fence. Just keep walking, with the water on your left, for as long as it interests you. The only choices along the way are to go forward, turn around, or exit at one of the other two gates.

As you go, you will find a series of interesting features on your left. The first is the dominant Hollywood Sign, which used to read "Hollywoodland." This was an advertisement for a realty company based in nearby Beachwood Canyon. The sign's last four letters were removed when the sign became the property of the city and, eventually, a world-famous symbol of the district.

Also on this hillside, below the Hollywood Sign, note the unusual presence of Hollywood's only commercial vineyard. The grapevines you see clinging to the high hills belong to the Hollywood Classic Vineyard. I'm told the winery produces a robust red wine from these grapes. Cases are sold by subscription only; those lucky enough to get on the list can expect to pay more than $100 a bottle.

The six-acre vineyard was founded in 2001 by Kenneth York, and was the site of a battle between York and his neighbors after he announced plans to expand his holdings to include a large house with wine "caves" and a tennis court. The neighbors protested, and the plan remains on hold.

Also visible from below is another storied piece of real estate. To the right of the vines is a cream-colored campanile, which is attached to the home once occupied by the Hollywood gangster Bugsy Siegel. According to legend, the house was home to a speakeasy during Prohibition. More recently, it was home to pop singer Madonna, who painted the house in gaudy colors and drew crowds of fans to the stretch of Mulholland Highway (named after William Mulholland) above the reservoir.

Walk on. Enjoy the shade provided by pine, eucalyptus and oak trees. Watch for animals, too—I have seen deer and coyote along the edge of the reservoir.

In time, you will come out of the shade to a straight stretch of walkway. Ahead of you is the dam itself. A peek over the side will reveal some of the less-visible artistry of Lake Hollywood. The front of the dam is decorated with the carved stone heads of California grizzly bears—the state animal, featured on the California state flag.

The reservoir was designed to hold 2.5 billion gallons of water, but it only held that volume for its first four years. In 1928, another Mulholland water project, the Saint Francis Dam in northern L.A. county's San Francisquito Canyon, collapsed, killing more than 600 people. Mulholland determined that it was safer for the Lake Hollywood reservoir to be maintained at a lower level. It has been kept at about one-third capacity ever since.

It's not uncommon to see film, TV, and fashion shoots in session here, on top of the dam. If you come across one, hang around, attempt to be discovered, and then continue walking around the lake.

It is said that Mulholland Highway used to run across the top of this dam, too. A length of it does come down the hill nearby, and the other side of it does continue not far away. But I've yet to determine whether this is true.

Just on the other side of the dam, you'll find a second entrance/exit, this one on Weidlake Drive. Continue to walk around the lake, in and out of the shade. After another stretch of quiet strolling, you will come to the lake's last gate, known as Tahoe Gate. Once you pass through this, you are out of the lake's enclosure, and back on city streets—actually, back on Lake Hollywood Drive. Cross to the right side of the roadway, and use the dirt pathway to continue your journey.

You'll get views from here of downtown Hollywood, as well as a different perspective on the mountains. There is usually little traffic along this windy stretch of road, but keep to the pathway just the same—there is no sidewalk.

In a bit, you'll find your way back around to Gate 2. You have circumnavigated the lake, and are back at your starting point.

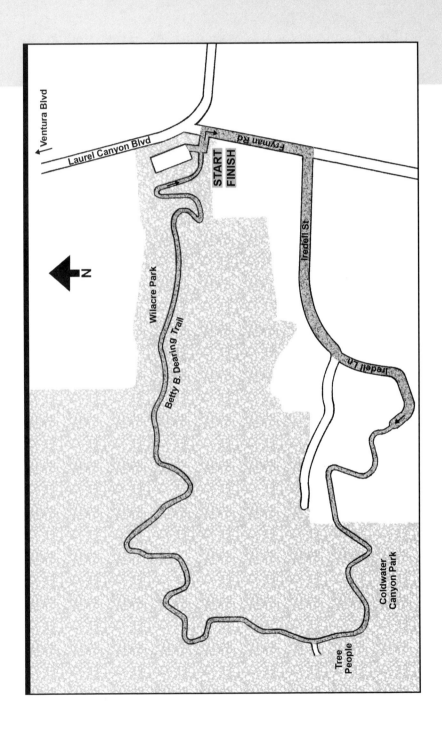

WALK #15

FRYMAN CANYON
DISTANCE: **3 miles**
DURATION: **1 hour 15 minutes**
DIFFICULTY: **3**
DETAILS: **Free street parking, and $3 paid parking. Dogs on leash allowed. Metro bus #218.**

This is a popular hiking and jogging trail that can sometimes feel too crowded, though it's not quite as busy as nearby Runyon Canyon. If you go early in the morning on a weekday, when it's quiet and the sun isn't so strong, you will have a better chance of seeing wildlife of the four-legged (not two-legged) kind. On the other hand, it's also a popular place to spot celebrities. Film, TV, and music stars abound.

Begin this walk from Wilacre Park, on Fryman Road a block west of Laurel Canyon Boulevard and about half a mile south of Ventura Boulevard. There's a free parking lot here, but arrive early on the weekends to find street parking.

Start walking south on Fryman Road, away from the parking lot and the trailhead. (That's against the flow of traffic. Most people will be headed for the base of a paved road going up into the park.) Follow Fryman under some oaky shade for about a block, then turn right onto Iredell Street. Another block on, under even more eucalyptus and sycamore shade and past some even more stately homes, bear left onto Iredell Lane (*not* right onto Iredell Street). You'll find the trailhead at the end of the cul-de-sac straight ahead.

This is the Betty B. Dearing Trail, a cross-mountain path that connects Fryman Canyon to Coldwater Canyon Park and extends up behind you to the Gene Autry Ridge. This section

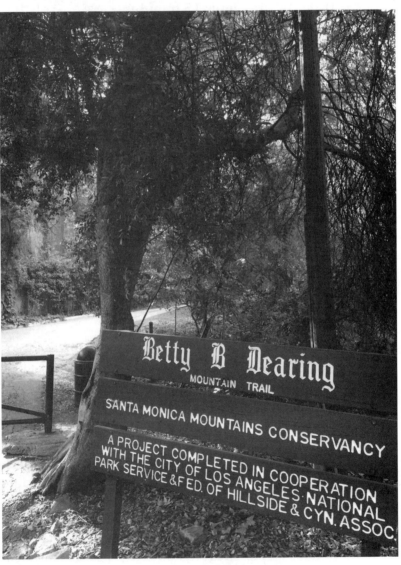

This former fire road was renamed in 1992 to honor
conservationist Betty B. Dearing.

of the trail is wide and dusty, climbing gently but persistently through an overgrowth of typical California flora: oak, eucalyptus, black walnut, and some scattered pines.

Walk up as the trail winds around, gradually gaining some elevation, and enjoy the views into Studio City and beyond. You'll find some of the best views as the trail flattens slightly and meets a spur off to the left. As signs will indicate, that's the way to Tree People, an environmental nonprofit that has been operating here for three decades. The facility is open to the public from 6:30 AM to sunset.

Take a break on the benches here, if you like, or walk over to see what the Tree People are doing. Then press on, continuing on the main road toward the ridge ahead.

The traffic may get a little heavier here. Along with the joggers and hikers, you may encounter mountain bikers—that's one of the reasons I like to do this walk against the flow of traffic, so I can see the bikes coming at me.

Stay on the wide dirt trail, avoiding the many thinner trails running off to the right as you go along. (One of these, the U-Vanu Trail, parallels the Betty B. Dearing Trail, and can be taken as an alternative route if you know your way and aren't concerned about getting lost. This path has less traffic and is a little steeper and more challenging in parts. You'll see it peeling off to the right as the Betty B. Dearing Trail begins its descent.)

The way down begins gradually, as the wide trail begins to sweep to the right and then winds through a series of gentle switchbacks down to the parking lot. Along the way, you'll get more valley city views and, perhaps, more views of hiking or jogging celebrities.

In time, the wide dirt trail will meet the U-Vanu Trail again, go through a final sweeping switchback, and turn into a paved road. Follow this down a final alley of black walnut trees until you drop down into the parking lot at the Betty B. Dearing Trailhead. You are back where you started.

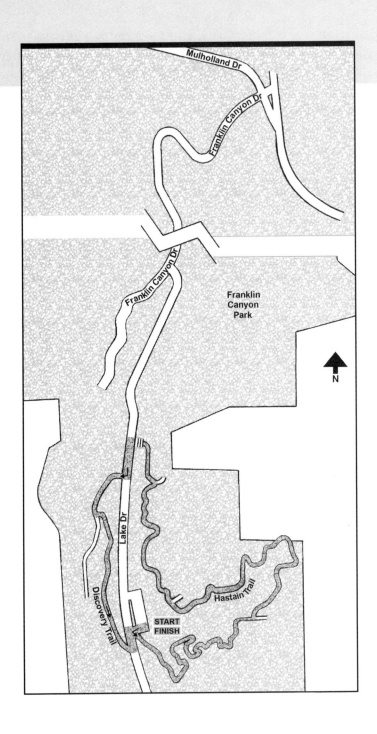

WALK #16

FRANKLIN CANYON RANCH
DISTANCE: **2.3 miles**
DURATION: **1 hour**
DIFFICULTY: **4**
DETAILS: **Free parking. Dogs on leash allowed. Park closed from sunset to sunrise.**

This unexpected location, hidden in a canyon south of Mulholland Drive, offers a classic Southern California combination: a dusty trail dotted with oak, sycamore, and eucalyptus, with dramatic city views. It pairs nicely with the Upper Franklin Canyon Reservoir Walk (see Walk #17) to make a really big hike.

Begin by driving south on Franklin Canyon Drive, heading downhill from the complicated intersection of Mulholland Drive and Coldwater Canyon Drive, or by driving north on Franklin Canyon Drive, heading uphill from North Beverly Drive and turning right onto Lake Drive.

If you come from Mulholland, drive carefully—making sure to really *stop* at the stop sign, since it's a photo-enforced, $100 citation if you don't—down the narrow lane to the parking lot on Lake Drive, about 1.2 miles below Mulholland.

If you approach from the south, come up North Beverly Drive from Sunset Boulevard, veer off to the right where Franklin Canyon Drive begins, and turn right onto Lake Drive.

In either case, you'll find the parking lot at the end of Lake Drive.

Walk to the bottom of the parking lot and past the public restroom. Then find the well-worn path that crosses the wide, grassy lawn before you. This is what's left of Franklin Canyon Ranch, a summer home built in 1935 by oil magnate Edward Doheny on land where his family used to graze cattle and horses.

Doheny was one of two important names in California's growth to leave their stamp on this canyon. The other was water magician William Mulholland, the man who designed the mighty Los Angeles Aqueduct and turned the city from a desert into a garden. In 1914, Mulholland oversaw construction of a dam and reservoir in Upper Franklin Canyon, one of many reservoirs he built to store the water he was sending (or stealing) from the Owens Valley to irrigate Los Angeles.

The path across the lawn is the foot of the Hastain Trail. Follow it through the grass, where you'll see a private home to the left and some sycamore-shaded picnic tables down to the right. Soon the path will tuck under an oak tree and begin to climb.

A series of dusty switchbacks will carry you past cactus plants and over a few sets of wooden stairs. It will hug the hillside and soon get a bit steep.

The payoff for the climb begins soon, though. Peeks at the Century City skyline and a small (but now covered) reservoir below give way to broader views that include Santa Monica, Marina Del Rey, the south bay cities stretching to Palos Verdes, and even Catalina Island.

The narrow trail will emerge onto a flat spot. Ahead and off to the right is a path that leads to the ridge above you—offering even better views, and a look down into Coldwater Canyon. This makes a good side trip, and a vigorous workout.

For now, or after that side trip, take the wider path that verges downhill to the left, staying on Hastain Trail. This trail will gently descend and go in and out of bits of shade, with views across the canyon. Along the ridge are some very stately homes. Just below the ridge, the line of elderly eucalyptus trees marks Franklin Canyon Drive, while the more colorful line of pepper trees marks a private driveway coming off Franklin Canyon

Drive near the southern entrance to the park. That's one shady driveway.

The trail will wind gently down, remaining wide, and will show the tracks of the mountain bikes that share this part of Hastain Trail. In time, the path will steepen a bit, and then flatten out for the last quarter-mile.

Hastain Trail spills onto Lake Drive under a nice bit of oak and sycamore shade. Drop down a set of wooden stairs and begin walking downhill on the road—but not far. After 100 feet or less, you'll see a sign for Discovery Trail. Cross the road here and pick up the unmarked section of this trail on the opposite side of Lake Drive.

The trail, narrow like the beginning of Hastain, hits an intersection just steps from the road. Take the left (or downhill) side and begin the gentle amble back down the canyon. This is a well-shaded walk through leafy meadows and under groves of sycamore, oak, and black walnut trees. It parallels the road, meandering between the trees and rising and falling a little with the landscape.

In time, you will catch glimpses of the parking lot where you started. Be patient. The trail will climb one last bit, and then deposit you back on Lake Drive by the southern end of the parking area. Cross the road, and you are back where you started.

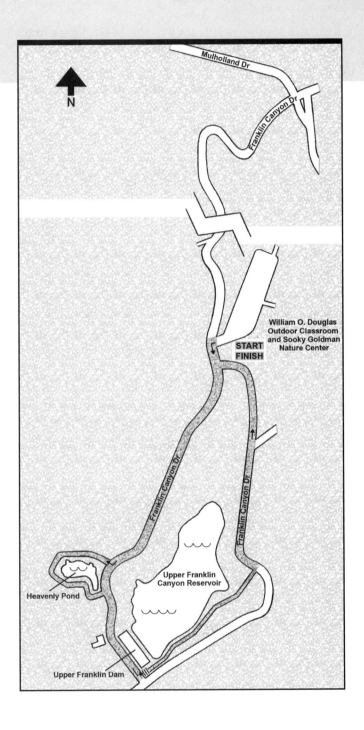

WALK #17

UPPER FRANKLIN CANYON RESERVOIR
DISTANCE: **1.2 miles**
DURATION: **30 minutes**
DIFFICULTY: **1**
DETAILS: **Free parking. Dogs on leash allowed. Wheelchair accessible. Park closed from sunset to sunrise.**

Here is a magical, hidden discovery: a pair of lakes right in the city, just minutes off the busy intersection of Mulholland Drive and Coldwater Canyon Drive. If you've never been here, but the area looks familiar, that's because it's been featured on TV and in the movies since the early days of Hollywood. It pairs up nicely with the Franklin Canyon Ranch Walk (see Walk #16) if you're in the mood for a bigger walk.

To find the beginning of this walk, drive downhill on Franklin Canyon Drive from the complicated intersection of Mulholland Drive and Coldwater Canyon Drive. (This street starts directly across Coldwater from the entrance to Tree People.) Down the canyon a bit, turn left into the parking lot for the William O. Douglas Outdoor Classroom and Sooky Goldman Nature Center. Watch out for the photo-enforced stop sign just after the parking lot! It's a $100 fine if you roll through it.

Just below you is the Upper Franklin Canyon Reservoir, where the history of this canyon begins.

Having already overseen construction of the aqueduct that

brought Owens Valley water to Los Angeles (see Walk #3 for more details), William Mulholland began building reservoirs to store that water. In 1914, he built one in Franklin Canyon to store drinking water for the citizens of the growing city below.

You can learn more about the reservoir's history at the Sooky Goldman Nature Center, just off the parking lot. Named after a local woman who was instrumental in saving the canyon from development, the nature center offers pamphlets and placards explaining what's going on around you. The center also houses an auditorium that features presentations on nature-related topics, and hosts free Los Angeles Audubon Society nature walks on the second Sunday of the month. There are also well-maintained restrooms and drinking fountains here.

To start your walk, exit the parking lot, turn left, and walk about fifty feet before bearing right onto Franklin Canyon Drive. (It's a one-way road here, so listen for traffic behind you.) The road will wind along, curving in and out of the shade of oak and pine trees. After a third of a mile or so, you will come across this walk's first water feature: Heavenly Pond, off to your right.

Although it isn't exactly clear what makes this pond heavenly, it is home to some ducks and turtles who seem to like it well enough. There is a path circling the pond, and benches along its banks.

Leaving the pond, return to the road, but consider walking on the other side. From there, you will soon begin to catch glimpses of the Franklin Reservoir itself.

This is where you might begin to feel some déjà vu. The lakeside here appeared in the opening credits of *The Andy Griffith Show*, when Andy and Opie are headed off to the old fishin' hole, rods in hand. (Go ahead, whistle the theme song if you like.)

But that's hardly all. This area was also used for scenes in shows like *Lassie*, *Bonanza*, *Matlock*, and, more recently, *Sons of Anarchy*.

This has been a movie set, too. The area was used for some of the country lane scenes in *It Happened One Night* (somewhere along here, Claudette Colbert stuck out her thumb, pulled up her skirt, and taught Clark Gable how to hitchhike). Heavenly Pond was in *On Golden Pond*, and the Creature from the Black Lagoon made its home in Franklin Reservoir.

Walk along with the lake on your left, as you round the lower end of the water and cross a bridge that is actually the top of the dam that's holding the water up. On the other side, if you want to extend this walk and connect with Franklin Canyon Ranch, take the trail straight ahead of you and then follow it to the right as it descends the canyon. A mile or more below, you can connect with Walk #16 from this book.

Otherwise, just before the intersection, look to your left and find some redwood steps heading down to the water's edge. (If you are traveling by wheelchair or with a stroller, simply continue around the lake, turning left at the corner and picking up the trail a little farther along.) This will give you a closer look at the reservoir and the birds that call it home—wood ducks and Mandarin ducks, according to the information from the nature center. Follow this path until it brings you back to the road, where a set of steps will lift you over the retaining wall and put you back on the road itself.

Bear left. Minding the traffic, which will be coming behind you on this one-way stretch of road, find your way back to the parking lot by the William O. Douglas Outdoor Classroom and Sooky Goldman Nature Center. You have completed the loop, and are back at your starting point.

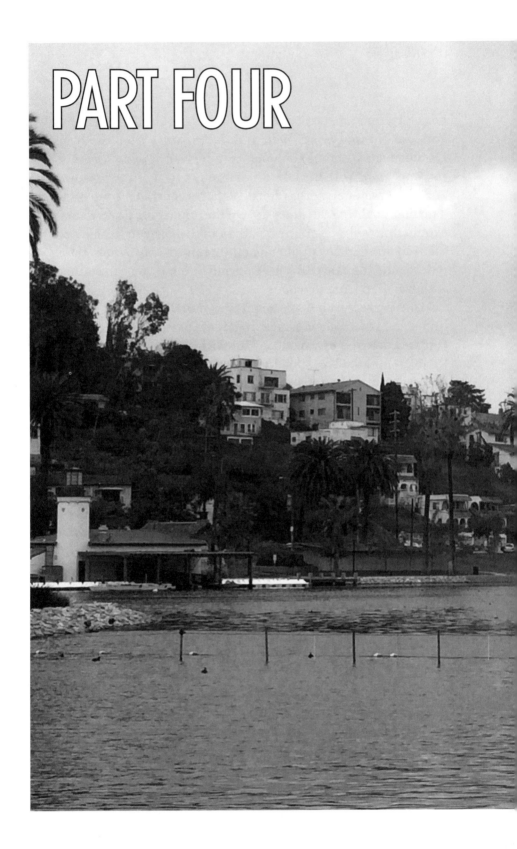

PART FOUR

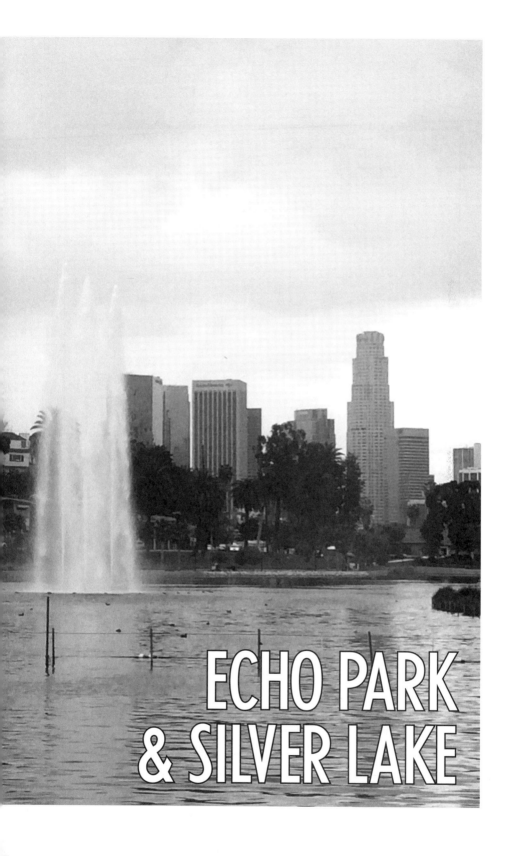

ECHO PARK
& SILVER LAKE

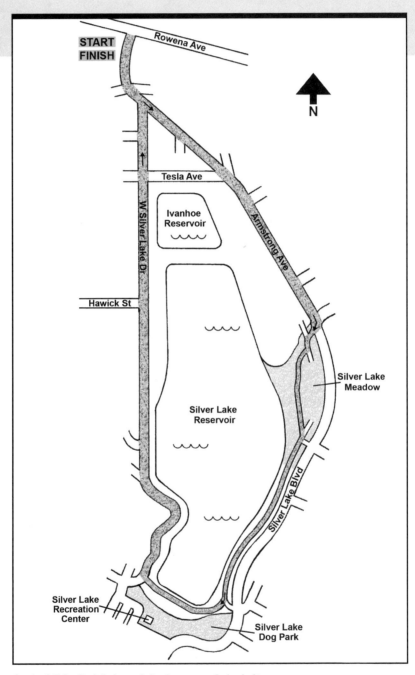

START
FINISH

N

Rowena Ave

Tesla Ave

W Silver Lake Dr.

Ivanhoe
Reservoir

Hawick St

Armstrong Ave

Silver Lake
Reservoir

Silver Lake
Meadow

Silver Lake Blvd

Silver Lake
Recreation
Center

Silver Lake
Dog Park

Overleaf: Echo Park Lake and the downtown L.A. skyline.

WALK #18

SILVER LAKE MEADOW
DISTANCE: **3.2 miles**
DURATION: **1 hour 15 minutes**
DIFFICULTY: **2**
DETAILS: **Free street parking.
Dogs allowed on leash
(except in the meadow itself).
Metro buses #201 and #175.**

This is a long, flat walk with almost no elevation change, circumnavigating the Silver Lake Reservoir and taking in the newly-minted Silver Lake Meadow. Popular with early-morning and weekend joggers, it's a nice, low-impact walk for anyone allergic to altitude.

Begin your walk near the intersection of West Silver Lake Drive and Rowena Avenue, perhaps after having a snack at Broome Street General Store (known for its hand pies and artisanal breads) on the south side of Rowena. Then set forth southwards on West Silver Lake, following this flat roadway until it meets Armstrong Avenue. Veer left, walking along a pleasant block of red-tiled houses shaded by flowering magnolia trees.

At the stop sign, where Armstrong meets Tesla, cross the street and get your first glimpse of the Silver Lake Reservoir, beyond and behind the Neighborhood Nursery School that is tucked into the corner of the reservoir compound. Step onto the decomposed granite walkway and begin to climb as Armstrong rises slightly, up and over a crest topped with pines, deodara cedars, eucalyptus, and oaks.

The wild property where all these trees grow is occupied principally by Department of Water and Power activities. But it is also home to a gang of coyotes, which can be heard howling at sunset.

As you descend, you'll meet Silver Lake Boulevard. Turn right, following the contour of the reservoir, and then turn right into the driveway that leads into the Silver Lake Meadow.

This is a new park area, achieved after years of infighting by local residents—some of whom wanted the land "preserved" for native species, and some of whom wanted a much larger part of the land around the reservoir open for public consumption. (The pedestrian pathways and park design are by landscape architect Mia Lehrer, whose firm also did the nearby Silver Lake Library.) The compromise: it's not huge, but it's open to the public, but since it lacks benches, picnic tables, and a parking lot (the space off the driveway is reserved for maintenance vehicles), the

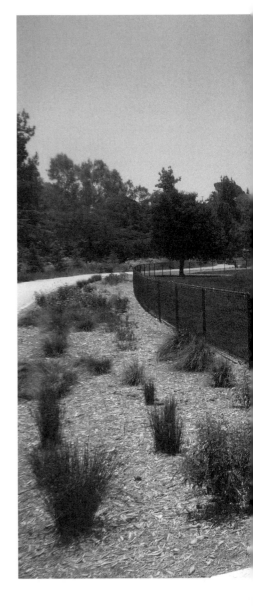

Peaceful Silver Lake Meadow, at the reservoir's edge.

public hasn't arrived in droves just yet.

Also, unlike the dog park just south of it, the meadow is off-limits to canines.

Nevertheless, it's a welcome green space, with broad,

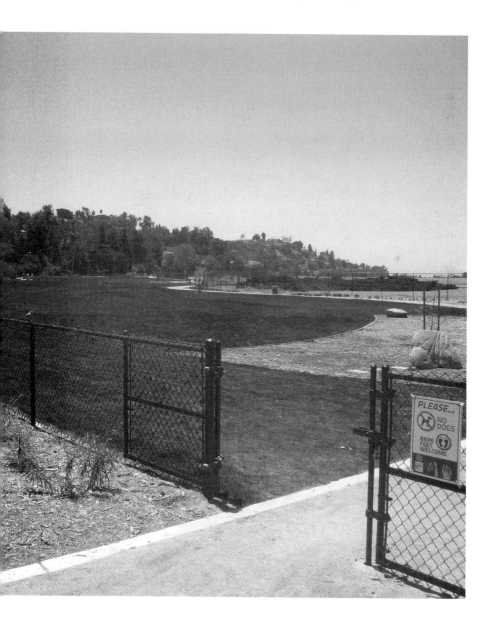

luxuriant lawns bordered by native grasses and trees that will be big enough to offer shade in about a decade. It provides fine views of two bodies of water: the larger of the two is Silver Lake Reservoir; the smaller is Ivanhoe Reservoir. The two basins' contents were once used to serve parts of downtown and South Central Los Angeles, but both were decommissioned and drained empty in 2007 after the water was found to contain high levels of cancer-causing bromate. The smaller Ivanhoe was refilled, and its surface was covered with shiny black plastic "shade balls" to prevent the recurrence of the bromate. The larger Silver Lake reservoir was refilled, but its contents are no longer used for drinking water.

Curiously, the reservoir is named not for its bright, shiny surface, but after the water commissioner, Herman Silver, who pushed the legislation that led to its creation in 1906.

Wander through the meadow. Architecture buffs will want to look across busy Silver Lake Boulevard to notice the modernist residences clustered there. Many are the work of father-and-son architects Richard and Dion Neutra, who, with Richard's acolytes Raphael Soriano, Gregory Ain, and Harwell Hamilton Harris, revolutionized mid-century home design. (The street paralleling Silver Lake is Neutra Place, home to several signature Neutra homes. There is also a Neutra home just across Silver Lake Boulevard from the meadow, almost directly in front of the crosswalk that more or less bisects the park.)

Continue on the pathway along the lake. Soon you will become aware of the sound—or the smell, depending on which way the wind is blowing—of the Silver Lake Dog Park.

Before you reach the dog park, though, bear right and follow the contour of the reservoir onto the new pedestrian path connecting Silver Lake Blvd and W. Silver Lake Rd. (The gate onto this path may be closed after hours. You can continue along Silver Lake, and turn right at the next corner, to circle around if the path isn't open.) Enjoy the clear view of the water here, then turn right, along W. Silver Lake. Pick up the decomposed-granite path, dotted now with ancient and newly planted redwood trees, and walk along the contour of the lake.

A long, straight stretch of roadway opens before you. When you get to about the 2100 block, look up and to the right and take note of the tall eucalyptus trees at the lake shore. Every winter, high up in these trees, small flocks of great blue herons build nests, lay eggs, and raise their fledglings, which are usually on awkward, leggy display in early spring. A plaque in their honor is posted where West Silver Lake meets a stop sign at the corner of Hawick Street.

You'll find a new pedestrian pathway on your right as you near Tesla. Step up for another close look at the water, or take a rest on one of the nicely-placed benches, and emerge at the corner

Follow West Silver Lake straight ahead until you meet Rowena Avenue once more. Turn left, and find your way back to your starting point.

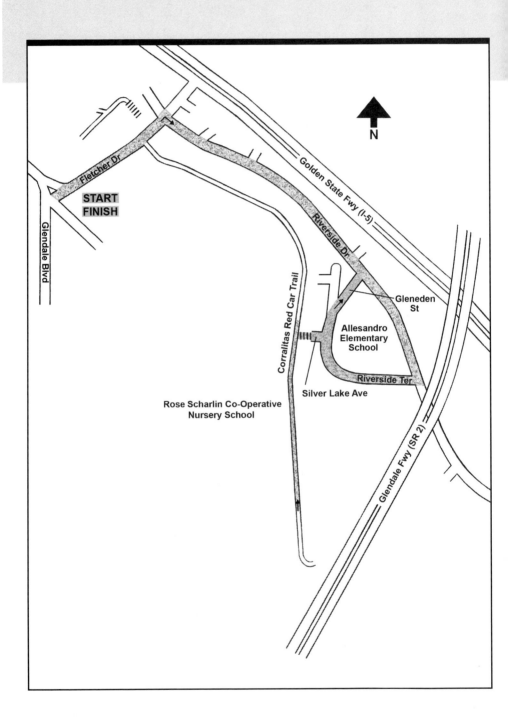

WALK #19

EDENDALE'S RED CAR LINE
DISTANCE: **2 miles**
DIFFICULTY: **2**
DURATION: **1 hour**
DETAILS: **Ample street parking.**
Dogs on leash allowed.
Metro buses #92 and #96.

Take a trip back in time on a walk that includes some surprisingly rustic sections of the hipster capital of California, including the remnants of Los Angeles's famed Red Car electric trolley system. Note that this walk includes one steep section. Wear good shoes and give it a pass on a rainy day.

Begin your walk at the corner of Glendale Boulevard and Fletcher Drive, perhaps after a coffee at the nearby Starbucks or breakfast at the Googie-inspired Astro Family Restaurant. Head downhill and east on Fletcher, with Astro on your right. Note the Apostolic Faith Fundamental Trinitarian church across the way (whose posted aphorisms have been a mixed source of inspiration and amusement for decades) and the Department of Water and Power's "City Water" building—a reminder of a time when public structures were designed with a sense of civic pride.

Slow down as you approach the corner of Fletcher and Riverside Drive. To your left, across the street, you will see a public staircase heading up the hill. On your right, you will see a series of concrete footings embedded in the hillside.

These are what remain of the Fletcher Red Car Viaduct, a

mighty trestle structure dating from 1906 that carried electric trolley cars from Edendale Station, to the right, across the river to Atwater Village Station, to the left.

The Pacific Electric Red Car trolley lines helped make Los Angeles a metropolis, and reached into every corner of the growing city. Lines ran east to San Bernardino, north into Pasadena and San Fernando, south as far as Santa Ana, and west to the beach and port cities of Santa Monica, Venice, Playa Del Rey, San Pedro, and Long Beach.

During its heyday (from about 1901 up to the 1940s) it was the largest interurban rail system in the U.S., running more than 2,100 trains a day over 1,000 miles of track.

One last impact on certain neighborhoods is the presence of . . . public staircases! Contractors and city engineers who were laying out streets in hilly areas designed the pubic stairways to help people get to the trolley lines from homes on steep hillsides. The roads may wind and bend their way down the hills, but the pedestrian stairs ran straight to the Red Car stations at the time.

The footings near where you're currently standing held up the viaduct, and the staircase took people up and down the hill, to and from the station. The trolley line was decommissioned in 1955, and the viaduct was dismantled in 1959. You'll get a better view of the trolley line later.

Turn right on Riverside and walk along the sidewalk, ignoring as best you can the roar of the Golden State Freeway (I-5). Notice as you go the remnants of stairs climbing up to the spots where houses once stood.

Shortly you will come to Allesandro Elementary School with its charming murals, some twenty-five years old, painted by the school children. This elementary school is one of the few in the city still served by a pedestrian "subway"—an underground passage to help kids cross busy boulevards like Riverside. The city used to have dozens of these subterranean pathways, but most have been locked or filled in.

Just after the elementary school, turn right onto Riverside

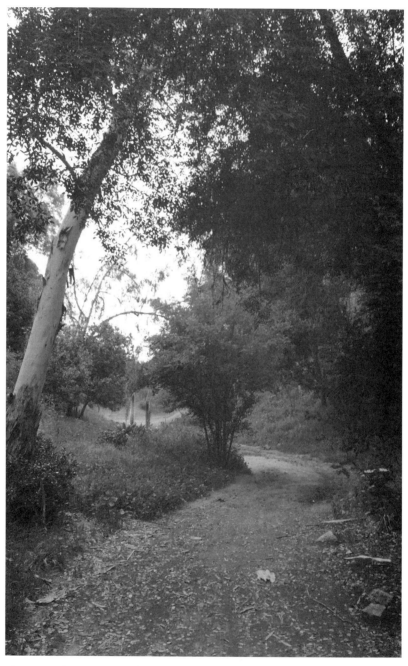

A section of shaded pathway that L.A.'s Red Car trolley system once passed through.

Terrace, and follow this as it curves up and to the right, behind and above the school playground. Then turn left onto Silver Lake Avenue, and walk a short block to a set of concrete stairs.

Just before that, note the strange Easter Island tiki heads in the house to the right of the stairs. I'm not sure what the story is, but I think they're adorable.

Climb the stairs and emerge onto a strange bit of Los Angeles—the broad, unpaved stretch of what's known on many maps as the "Corralitas Red Car Trail." This used to be home to the tracks that carried the Red Car trolleys from Downtown Los Angeles through Edendale (where you're standing), out over the Fletcher Viaduct you walked past a few minutes ago, and on across the L.A. River into Atwater and beyond.

For decades this has been an open space for hikers, joggers and dog walkers. Lately, though, it has inched closer to some sort of development. Enjoy it while you can by walking to your left toward a wide gate (which is almost always open) leading into a lovely shaded bower.

To the right, just before the gate, is Rose Scharlin Co-Operative Nursery School. Opened in 1939, this is one of the city's oldest private institutions. Walk past this and continue into a canyon shaded by black walnut, eucalyptus, and pepper trees. Go as far as the fences will allow, enjoying some of the peace and quiet of a clear, undeveloped piece of land.

Within the shaded area, you might look uphill on both sides, where you can see remnants of old public staircases that helped residents get down to the Red Car platforms.

Once you've taken in all of this, retreat back to the staircase that brought you past the tiki heads. Up to the left, you'll see more public stairs, also designed to get people down to the Red Car line. Straight ahead, you'll find more open land—at least until the developers develop it. Walk on and explore. You can go as far as a bluff above the intersection of Fletcher and Riverside, where you can appreciate the engineering required to run the Fletcher Red Car Viaduct to the opposite hillside.

Gazing off to the right from the stairs across Fletcher, you can see the expansive greens of Forest Lawn's Glendale outpost. Nearer at hand, you can spot the section of the L.A. River that the Red Car had to cross to get into Atwater Village—and beyond, since the trolleys that ran through here used to travel to the communities of Glendale and Burbank.

When you've enjoyed all that, retrace your steps back along the Red Car Trail. Look for the stairs you climbed earlier, coming in on your left, and descend. At the corner, turn left, again onto Riverside Terrace. Walk as the road bends right and drops down a block to Riverside. Turn left, walk to Fletcher, and turn left again to return to your starting point.

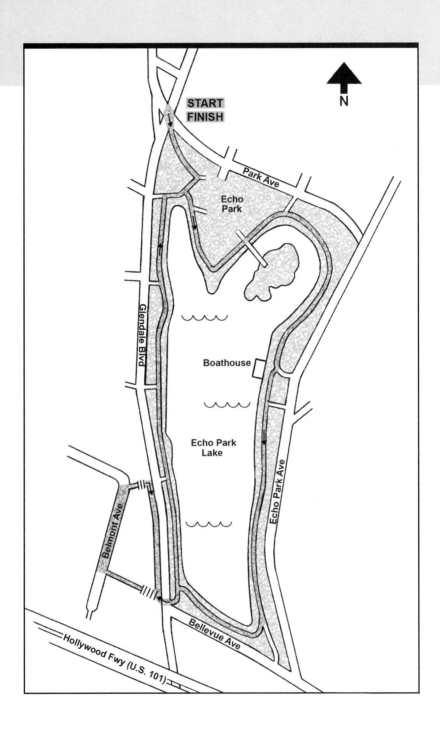

WALK #20

ECHO PARK LAKE
DISTANCE: **1 mile**
DURATION: **45 minutes**
DIFFICULTY: **2**
DETAILS: **Free street parking. Dogs on leash allowed. Lakeshore is wheelchair accessible. Metro buses #2, #4, and #92, plus Pico Union-Echo Park DASH.**

For years, Echo Park Lake was a seedy, depressing location with remnants of former glory, best avoided at night. After a recent restoration, it's now a popular garden spot—busy on weekends with picnicking families, guitar-strumming local kids, and sun-hungry old folks. The lake, its boathouse, and its signature lotus flowers are all back and better than ever.

Begin this walk at the northern edge of Echo Park, near the intersection of Glendale Boulevard and Park Avenue. Leave your car or step off the bus and enter the park through the thin, pointy end at that corner.

Already, you're surrounded by fascinating history. To your left is the mighty Angelus Temple, the vast 5,400-seat church hall from which Sister Aimee Semple McPherson established her Foursquare Church fame in the 1920s. Sister Aimee, a compelling public speaker, not only ran one of the Southland's largest congregations, but also one of the country's largest radio stations, broadcasting her sermons from coast to coast.

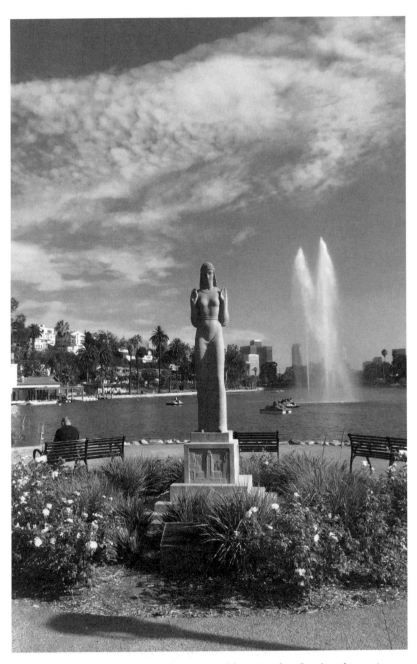

The Lady of the Lake, grounded by a pedestal featuring four Los Angeles settings carved in relief, including downtown's City Hall.

A Pacific Electric Red Car line once ran up and down Echo Park Avenue. Before it was discontinued in 1955, the trolley used to bring families to the church and the park. So did the electric trolley line that ran on nearby Sunset Boulevard, until it was discontinued in 1957.

Services still draw thousands to the church, which is now run in conjunction with the Dream Center. You can learn more about Sister Aimee at her well-preserved former home, located a block east at the corner of Park Avenue and Lemoyne Street. Free tours are given on weekdays.

Just inside the park, you'll find more history. To your right is a statue of Jose Marti, the Cuban poet and inspiration for the liberation of Cuba from Spain. The statue was placed here because some of those who fled another revolution—the one led by Fidel Castro—came to Echo Park and found refuge here. There used to be vestiges of this on the stretch of Sunset Boulevard running through Echo Park, once home to several Cuban restaurants. The Marti statue is almost all that remains of that community.

Now step into the park itself, and walk to the lake. At its head, you will see the beds of lotus flowers that are the centerpiece of the park's annual summer Lotus Festival. Canceled for years because the lotus flowers had died out, the festival is now back on since the park's revival.

Walk to the water's edge. Note the attractive skyline view of downtown L.A.—which you may recognize from the cover of this book—then bear left and walk alongside the lake.

The palm trees here are older than you are. Once a reservoir for drinking water fed by a canal from the Los Angeles River, and first designed as a park in the early 1890s, this space was landscaped and opened to the public in 1896. It included a boathouse, a community center, tennis and croquet courts, a pair of bridges, and these palm trees, and extended as far south as Temple Street—beyond the point where the Hollywood Freeway (U.S. 101) now slices through.

The lake has one specific vista point, and it's dead ahead. Here, stop for a minute to admire the Lady of the Lake. Added to the park in 1934, and originally known as "Nuestra Reina de Los Angeles," she is the work of artist Ada May Sharpless.

Beyond the Lady is the lake's fountain, and to her left, across the water, is the boathouse, built in 1932 to replace the original one. The structure was recently restored, and even the light in its tiny lighthouse began burning again.

Continue walking along the water's edge. You will see play structures and, most likely, food vendors selling everything from popsicles to bacon-wrapped hot dogs to corn on the cob.

On your right, you will see a footbridge leading to an island. Closed to the public for as long as I can remember, except occasionally during the Lotus Festival, this is now principally a bird refuge. You will see some birds sunning themselves and squawking as you pass.

Walk on and you will come to the restored boathouse, which has its own cafe. You can also rent paddle boats here—an excellent idea on a hot day, when the natural air conditioning of the fountain spray can provide very cool relief from the heat. You will also find public restrooms here.

Walk on and curve around the bottom end of the lake, enjoying the shade and creative landscaping. When you come to the next curve, take a few steps up to the sidewalk on your left, then use the intersection with Bellevue Avenue to cross Glendale Boulevard to the west. If you're using a wheelchair or stroller, stay on the pathway and follow the water around the lake.

Across the way, climb the public staircase up from Glendale, then walk up a wide, sloping path until you reach Belmont Avenue. Turn right, walk two blocks, and then turn right again as you come to a low white fence.

Here you will be rewarded with a fine view of the lake, the fountain, the boathouse, and the church behind the lake (to the right of the boathouse)—the seat of the Episcopal Diocese of Los Angeles. Higher up to the left and farther away, you can see the golden domes of the Ukranian Church of Los Angeles, too.

Straight before you are steps going back down to Glendale Boulevard. Take these to the sidewalk below, turn right, return to the corner of Bellevue, and cross back to the lake to resume your stroll. Turning left, you will find more lotus beds and other new landscaping to accompany the elderly palms and even a few scattered redwoods that remain from the park's early days.

In time, you will come to an elevated viewing platform fitted with benches. This is another great place to cool off on a hot day, or to admire the lotuses and the water birds that float among them.

Past the viewing platform, where there is loads of interesting information about the lake and its history, you will soon find yourself back at Jose Marti, Sister Aimee, and Park Avenue—and your starting place.

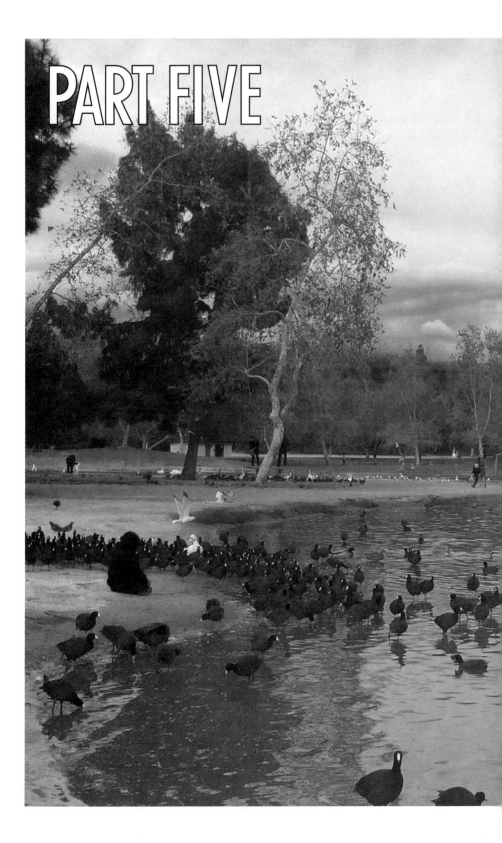

PART FIVE

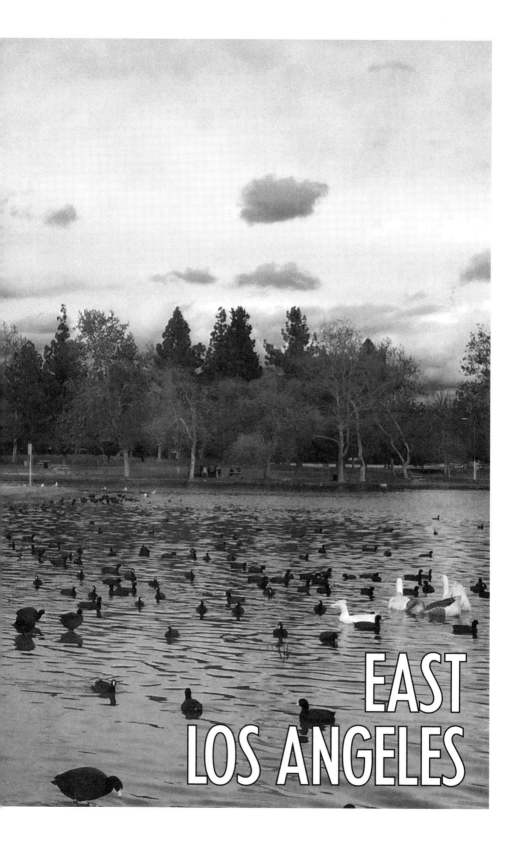

EAST
LOS ANGELES

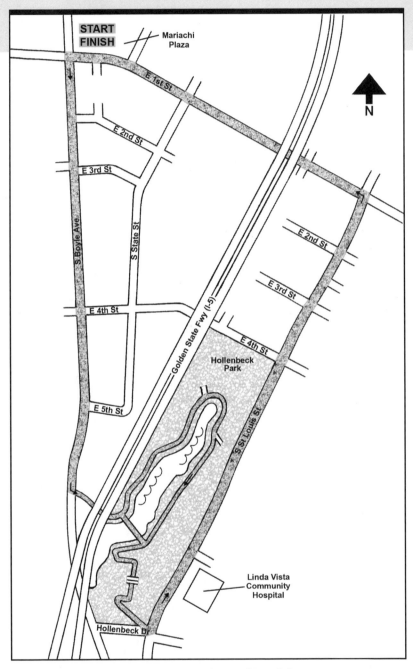

Overleaf: The Whittier Narrows Recreation Area and Legg Lake.

WALK #21

HOLLENBECK PARK
DISTANCE: **2.5 miles**
DURATION: **1 hour**
DIFFICULTY: **2**
DETAILS: **Free street parking. Dogs on leash allowed. Wheelchair accessible. Metro buses #620 and #30. Metro Gold Line, Mariachi Plaza stop.**

This walk is a gentle stroll through one of the city's oldest neighborhoods and parks. The extension of the Gold Line into Boyle Heights has made this part of the city more accessible, and helped create new hipster hangouts east of downtown Los Angeles.

Begin your walk at Mariachi Plaza in Boyle Heights, at the bandstand located at the intersection of East First Street and South Boyle Avenue, where musicians in their mariachi uniforms gather to wait for their next gig.

While you're at the plaza, take a look at Libros Schmibros—a combination lending library and bookstore.

Note the red brick building on the northwest corner of the intersection of First and Boyle. This is the old Boyle Hotel (also known as the Cummings Block), built in the late 1880s by an Austrian immigrant who made money in the Gold Rush. As one of the oldest commercial structures in the city, the hotel became a Historic-Cultural Monument in 2007, and has since been restored.

To begin your walk—and step further into L.A. history—start

heading south on Boyle.

This area is named for early L.A. landowner Andrew Boyle, who raised cattle here and grew grapes on the slopes going down to the L.A. River, across what is now the Santa Ana Freeway (U.S. 101). Boyle's former home, which overlooked the L.A. River from the bluffs above, was on the site of what is now the Keiro Retirement Home. The structure is gone now, but you will glimpse other homes from around the same period on your right as you pass Second, Third, Fourth, and Fifth Streets.

Of particular note on the east side of the street are the Neighborhood Music School at 358 Boyle, the Max Factor house at 432 Boyle, and the Elmer Simons home at 504 Boyle. The music school was established on this site in 1914, and has been offering lessons ever since. Max Factor, who grew up here, went on to become the most famous name in movie makeup. Elmer Simons's family operated the Pacific Brick Company, which built its wealth fabricating the building materials for the construction of early downtown Los Angeles.

The most magnificent of the homes along this road is another retirement home, Hollenbeck Palms, on the west side of the street at 573 Boyle. This immense building was first the residence of businessman John Hollenbeck and his wife, Elizabeth. (The family's Hollenbeck Hotel used to stand at Second and Broadway in downtown.) When John died, Elizabeth deeded her home for the creation of a home for the aged, and declared that a portion of the family land be used for the creation of a nearby public park.

Inside Hollenbeck Palms is a chapel that the Hollenbecks built in honor of their only child, who died as a boy. It now functions as a chapel for the retirement home.

Now cross back to the eastern side of Boyle as the street begins to slope downward and dip under the freeway. At your first opportunity, turn left and enter Hollenbeck Park.

Begun in 1892 with funds from the widow Hollenbeck, this twenty-one-acre park's central feature is the artificial lake you see spreading before you. Walk around the left side of the water

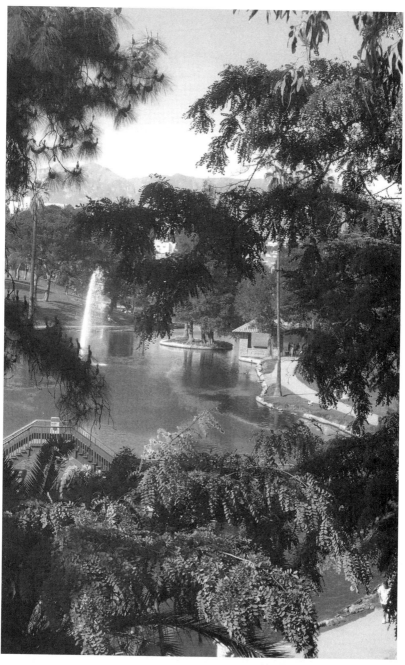

A glimpse of Hollenbeck Park Lake through the trees.

on the concrete path, and emerge from under the freeway and onto the park grounds.

The lake once featured a series of pathways and bridges over it. Now, only one remains—the footbridge on your right. Walk past this for now, circling around the western edge of the water. You'll pass sloping lawns, sometimes overrun by Canada geese, and some exercise equipment built by the city to encourage park visitors to stay fit.

Walk on, observing the island where ducks and geese gather under some redwood trees, and curve around the northern part of the lake, staying close to the water.

As you round the top of the lake and begin walking south again, you will see a few civic structures on your left, as well as some public restrooms. Along the water's edge is what's left of an old boathouse. (Like the lake at Echo Park, where the boathouse has recently been restored to working order, Hollenbeck used to offer boat rentals.)

Shortly you will pass the bridge again, which is a good place to stop and take a snapshot of the lake. Then continue on until you see a set of stairs climbing up to the left. Take these to the top of the hill—the high point of the park—for great views of downtown and the park itself. (If you're unable to take the stairs, stay on the main path and follow it as it gradually bends left and climbs up to St. Louis Street.)

From here, you can appreciate the varied greenery of the place. Over the years, the park's redwoods have been joined by pine, palm, jacaranda, eucalyptus, magnolia, and several kinds of oak. More recently, the park has added a small skate area.

The street behind the top of the park is South St. Louis Street. Across it, you may note a large, somewhat faded building that looks like a hospital. It is, or rather it was, the Linda Vista Community Hospital. Originally known as the Santa Fe Railroad Hospital, the structure dates from 1904 and was first built for rail workers. At its opening, the 150-bed facility had its own farm, with cows, chickens, and vegetable gardens sufficient to feed its patients.

The railroad later sold the hospital, and it was renamed Linda Vista, only to close again in 1991. Said to be haunted, in 2015 the facility was turned into senior housing and trendy lofts. Prior to that, it functioned largely as a TV and movie set. The shows *E.R.*, *Buffy the Vampire Slayer*, *True Blood*, *Criminal Minds*, and *NCIS* were shot here, as were some hospital scenes from the movies *Pearl Harbor*, *Outbreak*, and *In the Line of Fire*.

Turn left, facing the hospital, and walk along the top side of the park for a bit. In time, you will see a sidewalk sloping down toward a bandshell, where live music is sometimes performed on the weekends.

For your return, continue along South St. Louis, heading north once more, back across Fourth, Third, and Second Streets, through a neighborhood that features some charming period homes.

When you get to First Street, turn left and walk the two blocks back to Mariachi Plaza and your starting point.

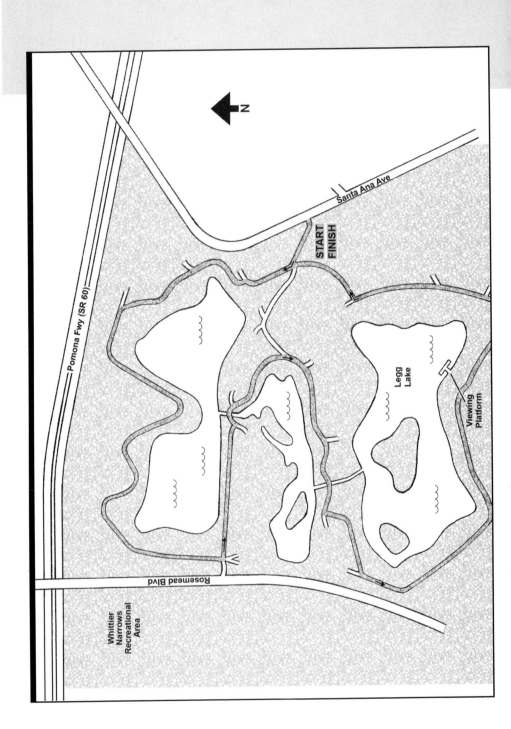

WALK #22

LEGG LAKE & WHITTIER NARROWS
DISTANCE: **3 miles**

DURATION: **1 hour 15 minutes**

DIFFICULTY: **2**

DETAILS: **Free parking on weekdays, and in some lots on weekends; $6 on weekends and holidays. Dogs on leash allowed. Wheelchair accessible. Metro buses #266 and #269.**

The Whittier Narrows Recreation Area is a 1,500-acre park that offers everything from hiking to golfing to skeet shooting. This figure-eight walk follows a flat, gentle route circling three small lakes and offering good views of the water and some interesting waterfowl.

Start your walk at the northeastern edge of this big open space off Santa Anita Avenue, just south of the Pomona Freeway (SR 60), from Parking Lot D, which generally does not charge for parking. You'll see the lakes before you and a concession stand renting bicycles. Walk toward the water and pick up the paved path heading off to the right. Follow the path as it loops around the northern end of the lake.

People who are familiar with Whittier Narrows mostly know it as the epicenter of a 5.9-level earthquake that rattled Southern California in October 1987. But the recreation area is an open waterway created by the convergence of the San Gabriel and Rio Hondo Rivers. The landscape may be man-made, but the water and the trees were originally there.

Circling around, you'll gradually bend left with the contour of the lake. In time, you'll pass a public restroom (identified as restroom #9) and a parking lot, and then you should see where the paved path runs between the northernmost lake and middle lake. Take this path and walk between the two bodies of water.

You may also hear gunfire along this stretch. That's because, off to your right, across Rosemead Boulevard, there's a gun club.

Walk between the two lakes, enjoying the pleasant sensation of water on both sides of you, and the shade provided by the area's sycamore, pine, and oak trees. Eventually you will come to a stone footbridge over the stream that connects the northernmost lake and the middle lake. Take the bridge, take the path to the right, and then bend slowly to the right and follow the contour of the middle lake as the path runs between it and Legg Lake, the southernmost of the three bodies of water.

In time, you'll come to another public restroom (this one identified as #7) and, behind a chain-link fence, a large dragon. (He and other great creatures scattered throughout the park are the work of artist Benjamin Dominquez. They are being isolated for restoration, it appears. You can see more of them at the Laguna de San Gabriel Nautical Playground in Vincent Lugo Park, in San Gabriel.) Pass a play area on your left and then cross another footbridge, over the stream connecting the middle lake with Legg Lake.

Keep walking until you come near the end of the water on your left, and follow the pathway going in that direction.

You may gradually become aware of a persistent buzzing sound. As you find Legg Lake coming more into view and the path begins to loop to the left along the shoreline, you will understand why—this section of Legg Lake is given over to radio-controlled boats.

Bend left with the shoreline, then stop (unless it's too loud) to marvel at the artistry and devotion of these RC boat people.

The ships are large and lavishly appointed. You may see ciga-rette boats, PT boats, or battleships trailered in from all over Southern California, manipulated by landlubbing captains out-fitted with complex guidance systems. They're fascinating to watch, and they make a huge racket, too.

Continue on, following the southern lip of Legg Lake. The noise of the RC boats will subside, and the water will become calm. As you get to the southernmost point of this section of the park, you'll find a viewing stand built over the water.

From here, you may see varieties of water birds, particular-ly a variety of ducks and herons, wading, floating, or skimming along the lake. (If you are interested in learning more about the animals of the area, visit the nearby Whittier Narrows Nature Center for displays and information about local wildlife.)

Follow the shoreline on around, gradually bending left and walking back north. Stay to the left, close to the water, as the paved path winds along and eventually passes a little waterfall where fresh water dumps into the lake.

You'll see a path separating the middle lake from Legg Lake, and one separating the northern lake from the middle lake. Take either of these paths to make a longer figure-eight walk or to extend your Whittier Narrows adventure. Or simply walk along the eastern shoreline, bearing right and aiming for the bicycle rental kiosk, and continue until you have reached Parking Lot D, your starting point.

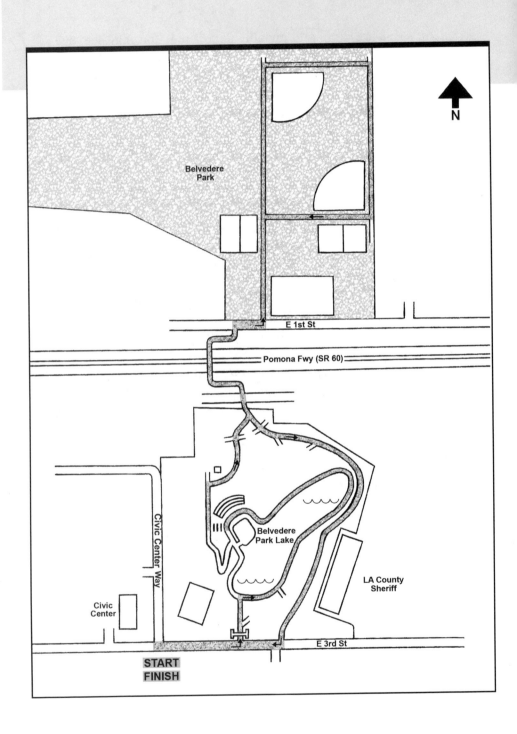

WALK #23

BELVEDERE PARK LAKE
DISTANCE: **2 miles**
DURATION: **1 hour**
DIFFICULTY: **1**
DETAILS: **Free parking. Dogs on leash allowed. Wheelchair accessible. Metro Gold Line, East L.A. Civic Center Station; Metro buses #258 and #68. Park closed from sunset to sunrise.**

This is another urban oasis—a green space built around a charming duck-dotted lake, shaded with a wide variety of native and non-native trees. The walk is freeway-close, and easy to find using public transportation.

Begin this walk at the corner of East Third Street and Civic Center Way, near the East L.A. Civic Center Station of the Metro Gold Line. Walk east on Third from Civic Center Way, then turn in between two colorful tiled gates reading "East L.A. Civic Center" and make your way down a slight slope toward a sweet little kidney-bean-shaped lake.

The civic center includes a public library and Probation Department building on the left, and a sheriff's substation on the right. Maybe that's why it feels so clean and orderly here. The only litter you'll see is probably what's been left there by the ducks.

And what ducks! So many, and so many varieties, honking

and squawking and gliding across the lake, and gathering at the feet of people who ignore the signs saying they shouldn't feed them.

At the lake shore, turn right and begin a circle around the eastern side of the water. Enjoy the flat concrete walkway, and the sight of two very big fish leaping up from the water at this end of the lake. In the late afternoon, the spray they create from their leaping produces a rainbow in the sunlight. (They must be rainbow trout.)

This is more than just plastic fish art. This lake is seasonally stocked with fish, and hosts an annual fish derby.

Far in the distance, if it's a clear day, you can see the San Gabriel Mountains. Though you are near both the Pomona (SR 60) and Long Beach (I-710) Freeways, you can't really hear the traffic.

You can also see that some effort and expense went into building and maintaining the park. The lawns are lush and the landscaping is tidy, using largely drought-tolerant plants. There are shaded picnic benches, play areas, and barbecue grills.

Walk along the side of the lake, staying on the sidewalk close to the water. Follow the shoreline until you come to an amphitheater on the right that faces what seems to be a floating stage in the lake. Musical performances here are common on summer weekend days.

Just past the amphitheater, take the staircase up to the right (or take the ramp, just a little farther around the shoreline) up to a parking level. Go right, and walk past a set of public restrooms. Bear right onto another narrow concrete walkway, roughly aiming for the pedestrian overpass up ahead, passing as you go a hillside boasting pine, sycamore, liquidambar, and even a few redwood trees.

Take this unusual pedestrian walkway over the now-roaring traffic to cross the Pomona Freeway to the other half of Belvedere Park. On the other side, facing the very attractive old Morris K. Hamasaki Elementary School, use the crosswalk to cross East First Street. Go right for about thirty feet, then turn left into the park.

On both sides of you are large shaded picnic areas. On the far right is the park's Aquatic Center—the pride of former assemblywoman, city council person, and county supervisor Gloria Molina. Walk straight ahead, toward a pair of tennis courts, and pass between them and a play area on your right. Then go up a slight rise past another set of public restrooms.

Here you will find yourself on a wide plain with baseball fields to the right and a soccer field and even a skate park to the left. If it is a weekend afternoon, the soccer fields are likely to be very busy. Spectate, if you like, then walk on, just past the baseball diamond on your right. Turn right and follow the sidewalk as it curves around the third-base side of the field. Walk until you run out of sidewalk, then turn in through a gate in the high fence and walk along the deep left-field side of the baseball diamond.

Here again, it is green and leafy and quiet. The noise of the park and the freeway will subside. You may be tempted to sit down on the grass and have a picnic. Go for it.

Walk until you pass a second baseball field, then turn in to the right, walking between the field and a set of basketball courts. You can also get an overlook of the Aquatic Center, which is open to the public year-round and offers free swim times on weekday and weekend afternoons. (There are also paid periods, offering events like "Senior Aquatic Aerobics," "Senior Lounge," and "Novice Diving.")

Continue on the path between the baseball diamond and the basketball courts, then walk down a slight slope toward the tennis courts. Turn left, and walk back to East First Street and the pedestrian walkway over the Pomona Freeway.

This time, once you're over the freeway, bear left and follow another narrow concrete walkway as it slopes down and bends right to give you another view of the lake—and perhaps a view of quinceañeras or brides and grooms posing for photographs.

Stay on this walkway as it follows the shoreline, but on a level above the walkway you were on a while ago. Follow along as it peels away from the water and crosses in front of the sheriff's substation, which is outfitted with a pair of stately Japanese stone lanterns (gifts, a plaque says, from the South Tokyo Rotary Club, presented in 1962 and 1964) and a line of "Safe Drug Drop-Off" bins (one each for prescription medications, "illegal drugs," and used needles).

The path will slope down slightly and lead you back to East Third Street, a little distance down from the colorful tiled gates that mark the official entrance to the park. Walk to your right, up East Third Street, and back to your starting point.

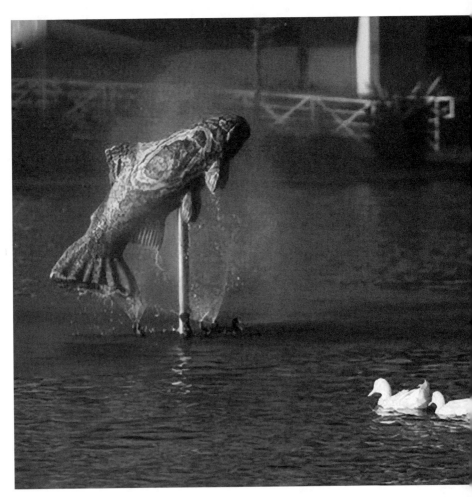

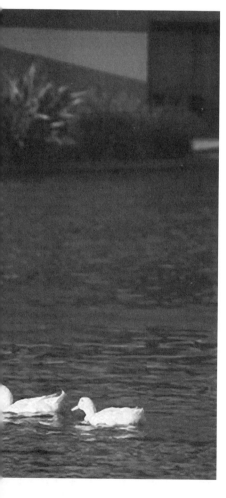

The lake's leaping "fish" promise waters well-stocked with the real thing.

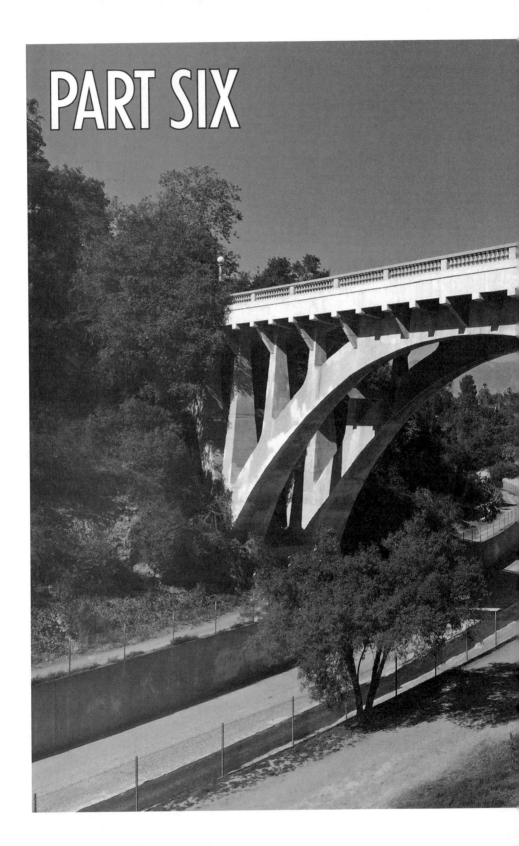

PART SIX

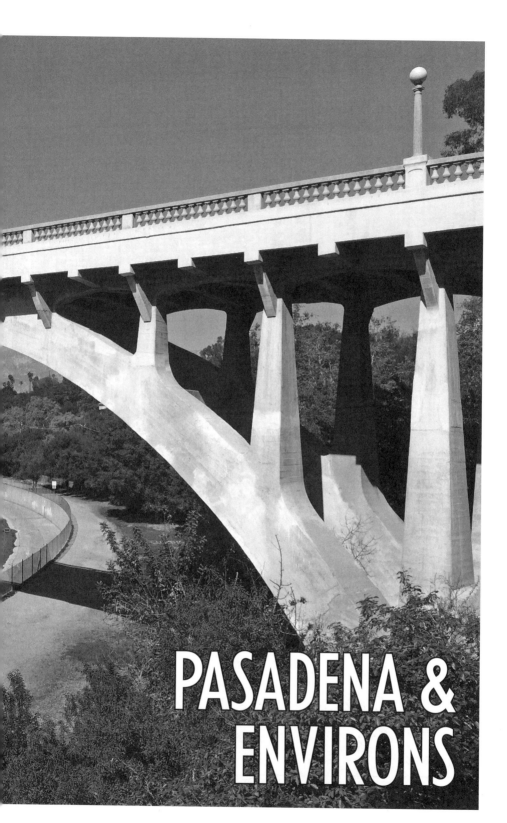

PASADENA & ENVIRONS

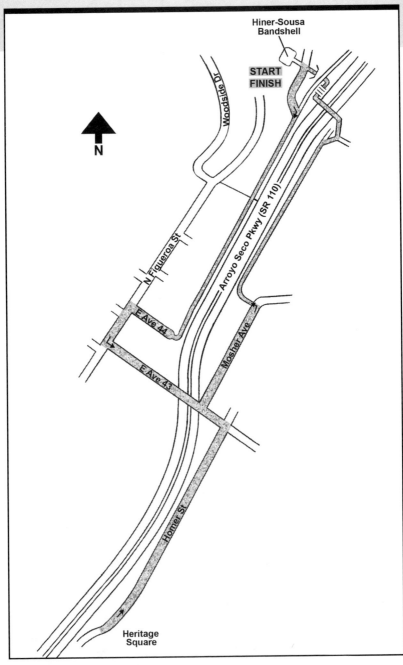

Hiner-Sousa
Bandshell

START
FINISH

Woodside Dr

N

Arroyo Seco Pkwy (SR 110)

N Figueroa St

E Ave 44

E Ave 43

Mosher Ave

Homer St

Heritage
Square

Overleaf: The San Rafael Bridge over Pasadena's Arroyo Seco.

WALK #24

SOUSA-LUMMIS WALK
DISTANCE: **3 miles**
DIFFICULTY: **1**
DURATION: **1 hour 15 minutes**
DETAILS: **Ample street parking.**
Dogs on leash allowed.
Wheelchair accessible.
Metro: Gold Line, Southwest
Museum; Metro bus #81.

Here's a gritty, freeway-close urban walk that follows the footsteps of two of early Los Angeles's most colorful characters: composer John Philip Sousa and writer/long distance walker Charles F. Lummis.

Begin your walk on North Figueroa Street in Highland Park, on the east side of the street near the intersection of Woodside Drive and a large, sand-colored bandstand. This is the Hiner-Sousa Bandshell, dedicated to the memory of the legendary marching band composer John Philip Sousa and his friend, Dr. Edward M. Hiner, whom Sousa visited here regularly. The Hiner House and Sousa Nook (used as Sousa's personal retreat) are a little north of the bandshell, on the west side of Figueroa.

Head south from near the bandshell on an asphalt path running under the shade of tall sycamore trees, keeping the freeway on your left. Walk to where the path turns right; veer left instead, and walk along a wide dirt path that runs close to the freeway.

That would be the Arroyo Seco Parkway (SR 110), formerly known as the Pasadena Freeway—one of the nation's earliest
highways, and famed in its early days for its forward-thinking
engineering and beauty.

You won't see much beauty here in this scruffy section, however, which sometimes functions as a hobo hangout and other
times as a public dump. Ignore the gang graffiti and walk on.

Pass the alleyway coming in on the right, then cross one
metal barrier and then another as the path narrows. When you
come to the next paved street, turn right onto Avenue 44, where
two beige apartment buildings stare at each other past a sign
that reads "End."

Walk past a few shingled Craftsman bungalows in need of a
little TLC, then turn left on Figueroa and walk one block to Avenue 43. Cross the street here, heading south, toward the Jack-
in-the-Box on the corner—noting as you pass the fine "grill
work" across Figueroa on the Family Dental and Orthodontic
storefront. Then turn left and head down Avenue 43 back toward the freeway.

At the first corner on the right-hand side, a block down the
road, you will come to El Alisal (generally translated as "Place
of the Sycamore Trees"), which is also known as the Lummis
Home. This is the hand-built residence of the restless, reckless
Charles Fletcher Lummis.

A remarkable man, Lummis was working as a journalist
in Cincinnati when, in 1884, he was offered a position at the
fledgling *Los Angeles Times*. Lummis took the job, and decided to
travel to his new home and workplace on foot—all 3,000 miles of
the trip, sending missives to his new employer all the way along.
Lummis later published a book about his journey called *A Tramp
Across the Continent*.

By the time Lummis arrived in L.A., he was famous and had
become something of an expert on the lives, culture, and habits
of the Southwest Native Americans he'd encountered along the
way. Making his home in the Arroyo under the alisal (sycamore)
trees, Lummis went on to become the city's chief librarian, and

helped found the Southwest Museum, later known as the Southwest Museum of the American Indian. The visiting hours for the Lummis Home and its grounds are Friday through Sunday, from noon to 4 PM.

To continue your walk, leave El Alisal and keep going east on Avenue 43, toward the freeway. On the other side of it, you will be faced with an interesting side trip.

Go two blocks on Avenue 43 and turn right onto Homer Street. Then walk about three blocks down to Heritage Square, a remarkable collection of elderly California houses and structures that includes a wholly intact soda fountain and pharmacy stocked with medicines. The buildings were all moved from other locations, and replanted here, and are in varying stages of restoration. (Hours are Friday through Sunday and most Monday holidays, from 11:30 AM to 4:30 PM. Entrance is $10 for adults, $8 for seniors, and $5 for children.)

Return to Avenue 43, turn left, walk a block and turn right onto Mosher.

If you don't care to see Heritage Square, go one block on Avenue 43 and turn left onto Mosher Avenue. Walk one long block to the park around Montecito Heights Community Center. Turn left at the parking lot before you get to the tennis courts and the baseball diamond. Look for a sign reading "S. Pasadena 2 miles," and follow this downhill onto the Arroyo Seco bike path.

Walk along this nicely shaded trail, which sits over the actual *arroyo seco* ("dry riverbed") below. When the path begins to rise and head to the right, take the pedestrian bridge on the left, and use this to cross both the riverbed and the Arroyo Seco Parkway.

Drop down two flights of stairs on the other side, then turn left and take the pedestrian underpass to return to the back of the bandshell, and the beginning of your walk.

If you want to enjoy a little more of the area, explore the nearby Casa de Adobe, Sycamore Grove Park, or the Professor's Row collection of fine Craftsman homes a few blocks north, along the Figueroa-adjacent Sycamore Terrace.

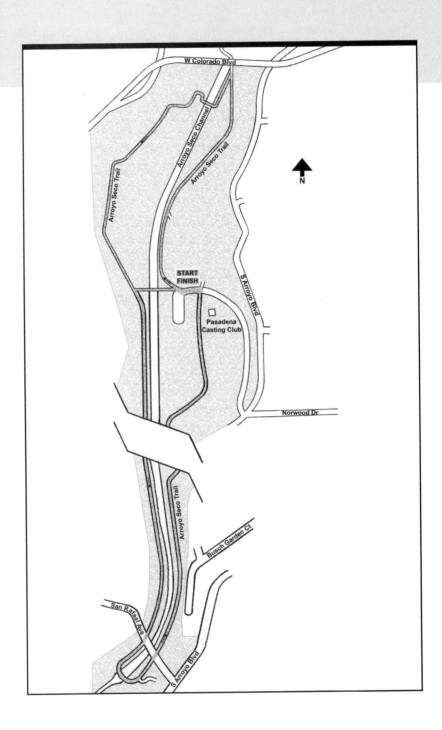

WALK #25

ARROYO SECO RIVER WALK
DISTANCE: **1.75 miles**
(or 4 miles for the extended walk)
DURATION: **45 minutes (or 1 hour 30 minutes**
for the extended walk)
DIFFICULTY: **2**
DETAILS: **Ample free parking.**
Dogs on leash allowed.
Metro bus #256.

Only a short distance from busy Old Town Pasadena and the rushing Ventura Freeway (SR 134), this walk in the country offers two options: either a short loop or a long loop, both full of bucolic pleasures.

Begin this walk just south of the Ventura Freeway and Colorado Boulevard, near the intersection of Arroyo Boulevard and Norwood Drive. Follow signs for "Pasadena Roving Archers" and "Pasadena Casting Club," and take the narrow driveway from Arroyo Boulevard down to Lower Arroyo Park. Leave your car in the parking lot and walk toward the footbridge to the left of the driveway.

Instead of crossing the footbridge, turn to the right just before you hit the concrete gulch that manages water flow down this canyon, and begin walking north.

Unlike the Los Angeles River, this part of the Arroyo Seco channel has not been allowed to revert to its natural condition. It's currently just a big, wide culvert, design to handle flood

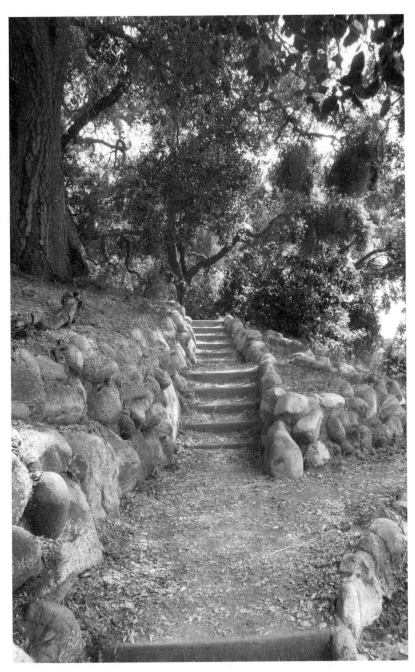

Remnants of the original Busch Gardens, once located here.

waters when it's wet and look ugly the rest of the time. Concentrate instead on the dusty path at your feet and the dense growth of pine, sycamore, and oak trees overhead.

Note as you walk along the elegant design of the Colorado Street Bridge, also overhead. The bridge, which got its name before Colorado was a "boulevard," is also known as "Suicide Bridge," for obvious, sad reasons. (The first person jumped not long after its 1913 construction. Dozens of others followed, despite the addition of a suicide barrier.) You may also catch a glimpse of the tiled, domed roof of the former hospital building on South Grand Avenue, now occupied by the U.S. Court of Appeals. In its heyday, this building also served as a hotel, and later a home for wartime troops.

On your left, you'll pass a pedestrian bridge crossing over the channel. Keep walking, and as you get right under the Colorado Street Bridge, climb a rocky slope to find the stretch of the river that *has* returned to something like its natural state.

Here the water is wide, and the plant life is wild. You can walk for about a half-mile up this stretch of the canyon before you pass under the Ventura Freeway and approach the southern reaches of the Rose Bowl area. If you come to a road, that's North Arroyo Boulevard, and it's time to turn around.

Enjoy a few minutes in the dense shade, ripe with the deep, creeky smell of slow-moving water and the sights of a wide variety of trees and shrubs.

Notice near the base of the bridge a marker indicating you are on the Tad Williams Trail, though the official name for the path you've been on is the Arroyo Seco Trail. This is a tip of the hat to a citizen who helped improve this area for walkers and equestrians.

Return the way you came, carefully making your way down that rocky slope, then turn right and cross the channel on the pedestrian bridge you passed earlier. Bear right, climb a slight rise, and then bear left and begin walking south along a wide path with some open creek to your left. Here again, there is ample shade, mostly from sycamore and willow trees, along a soggy patch that's busy with papyrus and cattails.

The trail will meander down and eventually meet the main arroyo channel near the pedestrian walkway that leads back to the parking lot. For the shorter walk option, cross the channel here and return to your starting point.

For a longer walk—and a treat—continue down the canyon. Turn right almost at once, onto the home turf of the aforementioned Pasadena Roving Archers. On a weekend afternoon, you may see as many as two dozen of the archers, bows in hand, pulling arrows from their quivers and loosing them at targets set along the canyon walls. Signs here remind you to stay on the path, and that's a good idea.

The path, marked by river stones, wanders through the archers' area under good shade, dipping back toward the main arroyo path before dipping away to the right and into the shade again. Follow this until the canyon narrows a bit and the path joins the main arroyo path again.

You'll walk under another stately bridge, this one supporting La Loma Road. The canyon will open again with a display of eucalyptus and palm trees on the right, and views of large homes on both sides of the canyon. (Locals might be able to tell you which one was "stately Wayne Manor" from the *Batman* TV series of the 1960s.)

As you cross under another high bridge, this one for San Rafael Avenue, take the narrow pedestrian bridge to your left and cross to the eastern side of the arroyo to begin the return journey up the canyon.

But first, notice the stone wall and steps climbing up to Arroyo and San Rafael. These stairs are remnants of some lost Pasadena grandeur. They are what remains of what might be Los Angeles's original theme park—the first Busch Gardens, built here more than a century ago by the beer tycoon Adolphus Busch.

On these bluffs, Busch built a complex system of fountains, streams, waterfalls, and winding walkways. In the early 1900s, this was his private garden, but the beer baron occasionally opened the grounds to the public. The gardens closed in 1938, but the theme park idea had stuck. Many years later, the beer company opened full-scale Busch Gardens theme parks here in Los Angeles and also in Tampa, Florida, and Williamsburg, Virginia.

The Pasadena property was used as a filming location for a while, but eventually fell into disrepair. But the streets to the right, where you can see houses behind a wooden fence, are still known as Busch Gardens Drive and Busch Gardens Court.

Walk on, up the canyon. When you come to two very tall, thick eucalyptus trees, turn right, following a wooden fence, and take the wide, sandy path curving away from the arroyo. Here there is more evidence, in the form of tracks and droppings, of horse traffic from the stables just south of the San Rafael Bridge.

Enjoy this path as it wanders through some shade and seclusion under clumps of old oak trees. Continue turning to the right as the trail meets the main arroyo walkway, winding toward the deeper shade. (Stay left at an intersection, though, where the trail to the right climbs up to Arroyo Boulevard.)

Keep walking. Where the trail brushes up against the main arroyo channel once more, stay to the right, keeping to the shadier stretch of path. Follow this a bit more, and come to the second of the area's official sporting facilities: a wide, rectangular casting pool (lighted!) for folks to practice their fly fishing techniques.

There are also shaded picnic tables here and, on the right, a small community building.

Just past this, turn left when you meet a road. Surprise! You are back at the parking lot and your starting point.

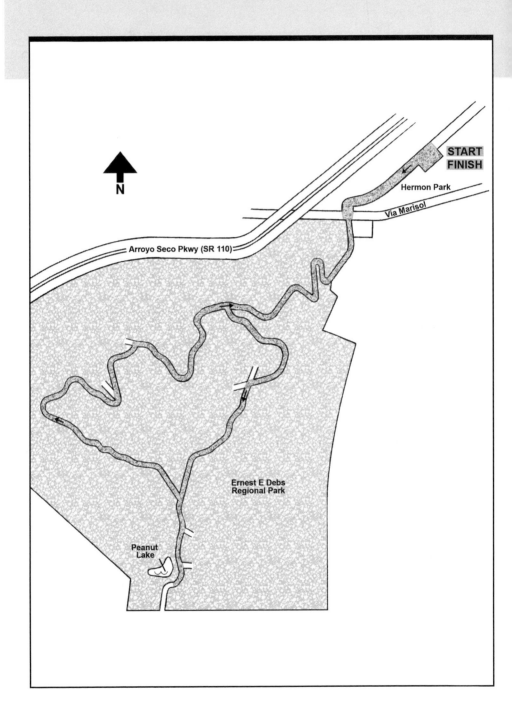

WALK #26

PEANUT LAKE & DEBS PARK
DISTANCE: **3.5 miles**
DURATION: **1 hour 30 minutes**
DIFFICULTY: 3
DETAILS: **Free parking at Hermon Park.**
Dogs on leash allowed.
Metro bus #256.

This is an extremely bucolic walk, beginning just steps away from the roaring Arroyo Seco Parkway (SR 110) and culminating in an unexpected water feature, high above the noise, and a lovely view of the downtown skyline.

For this walk, take advantage of the free parking, public restrooms, and drinking fountains at Hermon Park on Via Marisol, just east of where it crosses the Arroyo Seco Parkway.

Leave the parking lot on foot the same way you drove in. Across Via Marisol and past a steel barrier, you'll see a dirt road leading up to a set of old-fashioned metal gates. Walk up this road, and around the gates. You're on your way.

This wide dirt road will rise and wind for a while. Relax and enjoy the walk. As you go, you'll pass under oak and sycamore trees and see remnants of ruined dwellings—footings, bits of stairway, brick fireplace rubble—some of them decorated with graffiti.

Climb on. Gradually, the foliage will part to reveal bits of the scenery below. Here is the usually dry section of the arroyo's bike path and storm drain. Behind it is the Arroyo Seco Parkway, Los Angeles's first (and most scenic, and reputedly most dangerous) freeway.

Once upon a time, there was to be a different kind of freeway there. An entrepreneur impressed with the bicycle began a venture to build an elevated, wooden bicycle expressway from the Green Hotel in Pasadena to downtown Los Angeles. The cycleway, which looked like a fishing pier, included northbound and southbound lanes, exits, and toll booths. For a while, it even included bicyclists. But the cycleway didn't even make it as far as Hermon, the nearest town to the Via Marisol exit, before the idea fell into disfavor. Now, nothing remains of the cycleway but the dream.

You can probably also see, across the canyon, the lovely Southwest Museum of the American Indian, now controlled by the group that runs the Autry National Center in Griffith Park.

Where the road forks, bear left and continue walking uphill. In time, the dirt road will meet a paved road. Bear left onto the paved road, and follow it as the road descends and flattens and passes a wooden shade structure on your left. This is a good place to cool off, use the public water spigot, and look down over the eastern stretches of Ernest E. Debs Regional Park, which you've entered from the western side.

The 300-acre wooded park's main entrance is at Debs Park Road, off Monterey Road, one canyon over from where you're walking now. If you're keen to see it after this walk, drive up Via Marisol from the Hermon Park lot, turn right on Monterey, and drive about two miles. Debs Park Road will be on your right. The site also offers free parking, picnic benches, public restrooms, and water fountains.

Keep walking straight, avoiding for now another stretch of road running uphill to the right and several trail options on either side. The road will drop down, flatten, and rise again. Rise with it.

As it reaches its peak, you'll begin to see signs of human interference with nature—pine trees that probably weren't native to this area, concrete and brick footings, and, off to the right of the road, what looks like a series of pools.

Where the road forks to go around a slight promontory, bear right onto a dirt path. This leads to the charming Peanut Lake, also known as Debs Lake—a small but very charming body of water ringed by conifers and providing the most surprising views of downtown Los Angeles.

Locals I have met remember a structure that once stood on the promontory sitting over the lake—a hotel, some of them say, or a ranch house, with a view that went across the lake and toward downtown.

Now all that's left is the foundation, the lake, and a series of dry concrete pools where water once ran, bordered by walkways.

Leave the lake the same way you came, back on the dirt path to the paved road. For a much longer walk, you can turn right and follow this road all the way down to the main section of Ernest E. Debs Regional Park, take advantage of their facilities, and then come back to this spot.

For now, though, turn left onto the paved road and return the way you came, walking downhill gradually. You'll pass a little concrete building on the left. Shortly after, a dirt road will come in on the left. (If you've reached the shade structure where you stopped earlier, you've gone a little too far.) Leave the paved road for this dirt road, and begin making your way downhill.

This road will narrow to a path, and the way will get a little steeper. Go slowly. Down and to the left, you'll begin to see the structure and landscape of the Audubon Center at Debs Park. Open Tuesday through Saturday, from 9 AM to 5 PM, this is a great place to learn more about the region and its winged inhabitants.

Ahead is a slightly complicated junction. There are two roads bending off to the right—an upper one and a lower one—and a trail heading more or less straight ahead. The trail leads to the Audubon Center, so this is a good spot to include that in your walk, if you like.

Otherwise, take the second or lower of the two roads to the right (the one below the handily placed benches) and continue your walk.

This road will wind down and merge with another road, just

after some odd staircases that rise up into a narrow canyon on the right. Turn right onto this new road, and walk on. It will carry you along a more or less flat section, with trees and hillside on your right and some open field on your left. At the next intersection, stay right again (not on the skinny path straight ahead, but the wide dirt road to the right) and walk on.

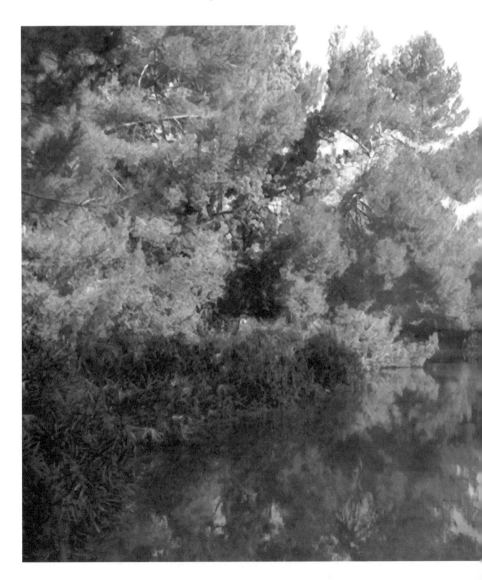

This section of dirt road will begin to rise again. In time, it will come to a peak and hit the dirt road that brought you up the hill in the first place. Bear left, and continue downhill until the road returns you to Via Marisol and, across the street in Hermon Park, your starting point.

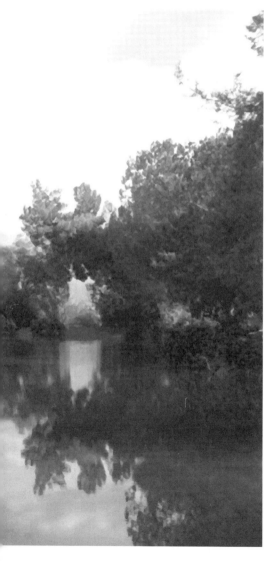

Peanut Lake is a placid, pleasant surprise at the end of this walk.

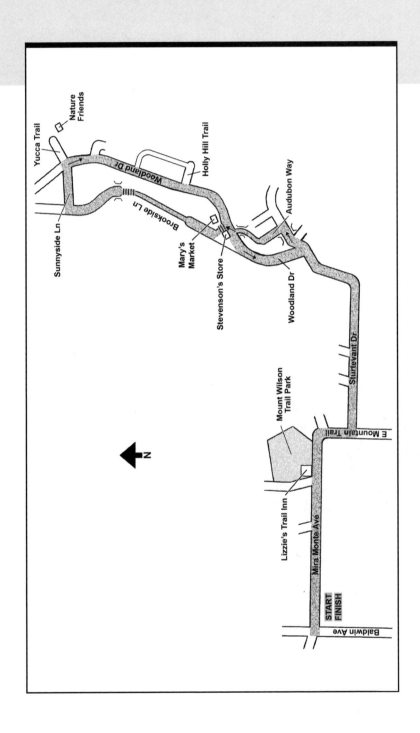

WALK #27

SIERRA MADRE STROLL
DISTANCE: **2 miles**
DURATION: **1 hour**
DIFFICULTY: **2**
DETAILS: **Free street parking. Dogs on leash allowed. Metro bus #487.**

This mostly pavement walk is a stroll into the past, when "The Great Hiking Era" struck the Los Angeles area mountains. If you pick the right time, your visit can also include a museum, a charming country store/restaurant, and a place that's been making jam for 120 years.

Start this walk in Sierra Madre, perhaps after a visit to the charming downtown district just east of the intersection of Baldwin Avenue and East Mira Monte Avenue. From there, observe a little history.

This is the traditional trailhead for the walk to Mount Wilson. It was once served by

During the Great Hiking Era at the end of the nineteenth century, this establishment helped outfit walkers for the climb to Mount Wilson.

the charming wooden structure on the corner—Lizzie's Trail Inn, which use to be the outfitter for folks headed into the hills. Today it functions as a museum, with fascinating photographs and artifacts representative of what was known as "The Great Hiking Era," when Californians took to walking as a hobby from the 1880s to the turn of the century.

After you've enjoyed that history—and perhaps even had a picnic next door at Mount Wilson Trail Park—walk downhill on Mira Monte, bend right onto East Mountain Trail, and then take a left onto Sturtevant Drive. Right away you'll begin to see bigger homes, under bigger trees, and begin to feel the magic of this walk.

Follow a freestone wall as Sturtevant bends left and then right. At the corner of Sturtevant and Woodland Drive, notice the curious sculptures made of ceramic pots on the left, then continue on Sturtevant to the right. Cross the creek using the concrete bridge, and then turn left immediately onto narrow Audubon Way.

This feels like a private driveway, but it's a public path. Walk on until it seems that the way has become blocked, but then turn left (following a hand-lettered sign for "Footpath") and cross the creek again on a narrow footbridge.

Now you're in the heart of historic old Sierra Madre. Directly in front of you is Stevenson's Store, where a brass plaque will tell you that this was once a store, lodging house, and tea garden. Just to the right of you, slightly uphill, is Mary's Market and Canyon Café, a charming place to grab some home cooking after your walk.

Head toward Mary's. Just before you arrive, though, look to the left for three stone steps and an asphalt walkway. Climb these, and after fifty feet turn left onto a very narrow street. This is Brookside Lane. Follow it as it meanders up the canyon, climbing slightly under big oak and sycamore trees. Just after the house at 570, the pavement will end. Walk onto a dirt path that narrows and climbs further up the canyon, with the creek visible below on your right.

Soon, you'll climb five metal steps and cross the creek on a metal footbridge. On the other side, under an immense sycamore tree, turn right and walk uphill toward an impressive covered wooden bridge. Past this, at the intersection, turn right onto Sunnyside Lane. Walk a flat block—again under impressive shade from a good mix of oak, sycamore, pine, and eucalyptus trees—before turning right and heading downhill on Woodland Drive.

Descend, enjoying the shade and the quiet. But first, notice on your left, at the corner of Yucca Trail, a sign for "Nature Friends." This is the L.A. outpost of an international nonprofit, born in Austria in 1895 and devoted to the love of the outdoors. Their Sierra Madre property dates from the 1920s and functions today as a retreat center, event space, and more. The group also hosts seasonal hikes and other activities.

Heading downhill some more, on your left you will see a house with highly decorated walls and, next to it, a sign for Holly Hill Trail. This is a semi-private pathway running behind the houses before you. To add an extra side trip to this walk, climb the stairs, turn right, and wander down a brick-and-railroad-tie walkway that leads back to Woodland.

Soon Woodland will cross the creek once more, and you will find Mary's on your right. Pause here for refreshments, and then continue on—past Stevenson's and past the ceramic pottery sculptures, to turn right onto Sturtevant once more. Follow this to East Mountain Trail, turn right, and then turn left onto Mira Monte. You'll find Lizzie's Trail Inn on the right, and you'll be back at your starting point.

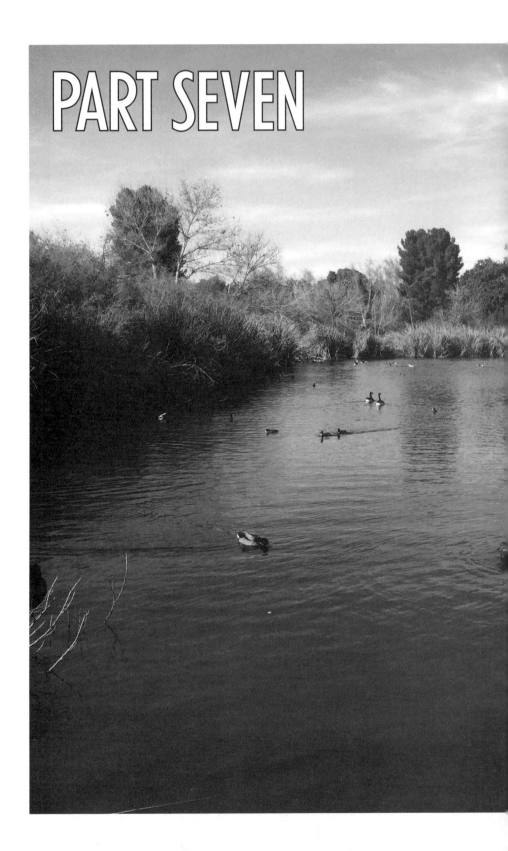

PART SEVEN

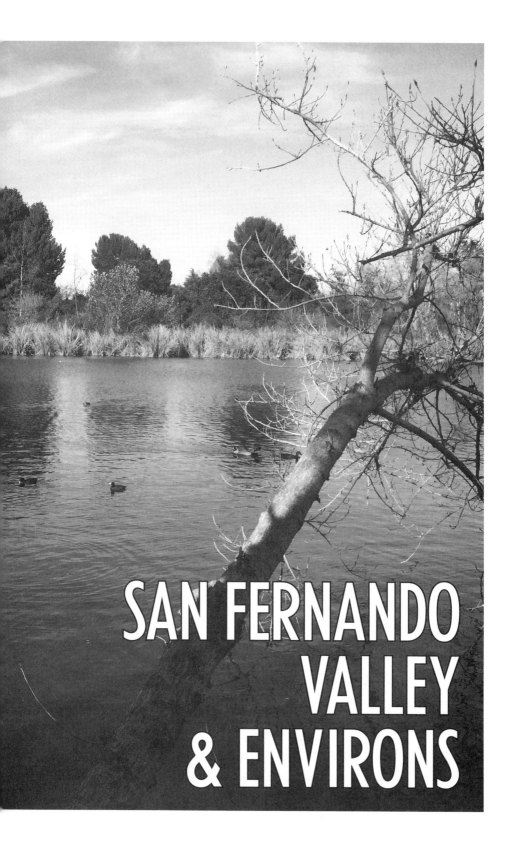

SAN FERNANDO
VALLEY
& ENVIRONS

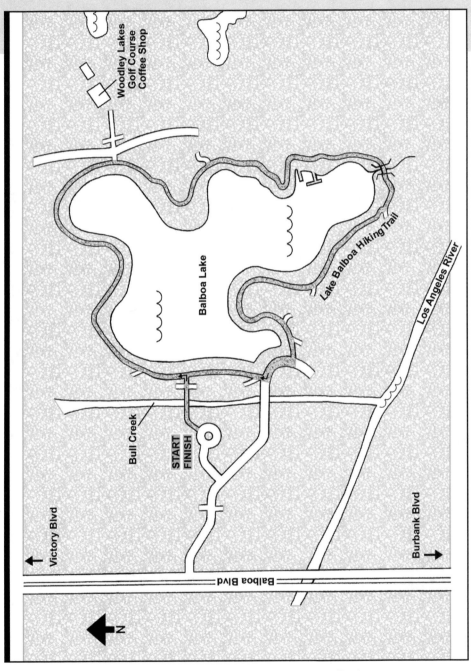

Overleaf: The Sepulveda Basin Wildlife Reserve is home to 200 species of birds.

WALK #28

LAKE BALBOA
    DISTANCE: **1.75 miles**
       DIFFICULTY: **1**
         DURATION: **45 minutes**
           DETAILS: **Ample free parking.**
                    Wheelchair accessible.
                    Dogs on leash allowed.
                    Metro buses #164, #236, and
                    #237, plus Orange Line bus
                    #901.

The San Fernando Valley isn't particularly known for its walking, hiking, or natural green spaces, so this unexpected oasis—in the Sepulveda Dam area, just minutes from the intersection of the Ventura (U.S. 101) and San Diego (I-405) Freeways—is all the more magical for its location.

Begin this walk from the western edge of the large Anthony C. Beilenson recreation area, entering from Balboa Boulevard about halfway between Burbank Boulevard and Victory Boulevard. Turn into the main drive from Balboa, then turn left into the very first parking lot you meet, an unpaved one. Leave your car at the left side of the cul-de-sac end of the driveway, then find the pedestrian walkway and follow it over the creek and up to the lakefront.

Beilenson was a Democratic congressman who represented the Southern California area from 1977 to 1997. He was instrumental in writing the legislation that created the Santa Monica

Mountains National Recreation Area and the Channel Islands National Park. The eighty-acre Lake Balboa Park was named in his honor.

Turn left onto the pedestrian walkway and begin a clockwise circumnavigation of the twenty-seven-acre artificial lake (which is filled by water that has gone through the nearby Donald C. Tillman Water Reclamation Plant, which also feeds the ponds and lakes of the delightful Japanese Garden). The air temperature may feel like it has dropped about ten degrees, from the cool breeze coming off the water.

The demographics may have changed, too; this is one of the most international parks in the city, a regular Tower of Babel of languages and cultures. If it's a crowded weekend day, you may see surprisingly varied clothing choices, and you may smell a wide variety of menu items if the park's barbecue grills are busy.

Ducks and other water birds dot the shoreline, as do fishermen. Although there is no fishing allowed in some areas—you'll know which ones by the posted signs—you may see anglers trying their luck on the northern shores of the lake. They are admonished, though, in several places by signs with messages like "No Digging For Worms Allowed." This may be the only park in the city that has such warning signs, or needs them.

For those not fishing, the lake is ringed by attractive shade structures, most with benches underneath, and many covered with wisteria vines.

The shoreline itself is planted with a mix of pine and sycamore trees with the occasional deodara cedar, all bringing welcome shade to the walkway, particularly on this northeastern side of the water.

Curling around the top of the lake, you'll note some wide grassy fields as the park stretches toward Victory Boulevard, great for pick-up softball or for flying a kite. Folks willing to walk a little farther can enjoy a more private picnic here, or stretch their hammocks between shade trees.

A cascade tumbles into the water at the lake's northernmost point—sometimes, anyway, but perhaps less often during drought periods. About 300 feet past that, if you're overheated or ready for a change, leave the lake path and head to your left. Cross the road, find a pedestrian bridge like the one where you started, and follow this over another creek, past a sign that reads "Woodley Lakes Golf Course."

On the other side and just to the left is a little shop, open from 6 AM to 4 PM, seven days a week, where you can buy a snack or cold drink to enjoy while sitting in the shade and watching the golfers on the putting green. There's also a pond that is sometimes busy with Canada geese.

Back at the lake, continue around the shoreline to a boat ramp and a dock that supports a more interesting collection of bird life. There are black cormorants here, keeping to themselves as if they had their own exclusive club, and a smattering of other water birds and ducks.

A stream flows out of the lake at its southern end, where the crowds and the barbecue smells grow thicker. So do the songs of the dueling ice cream trucks, placed strategically around the parking lot.

Past the stream and over to the left is a special enclosed baseball diamond for players with disabilities. Just beyond that, back at the lakeside, is a "flycasting area" for people to practice that other, non-Hollywood kind of casting.

Follow the walkway around the shore, past the busiest part of the park—where you'll find public restrooms and drinking fountains, if you need them—until you come back around to the eastern side of the water. Take the pedestrian bridge on your left to return to the parking lot and your starting point.

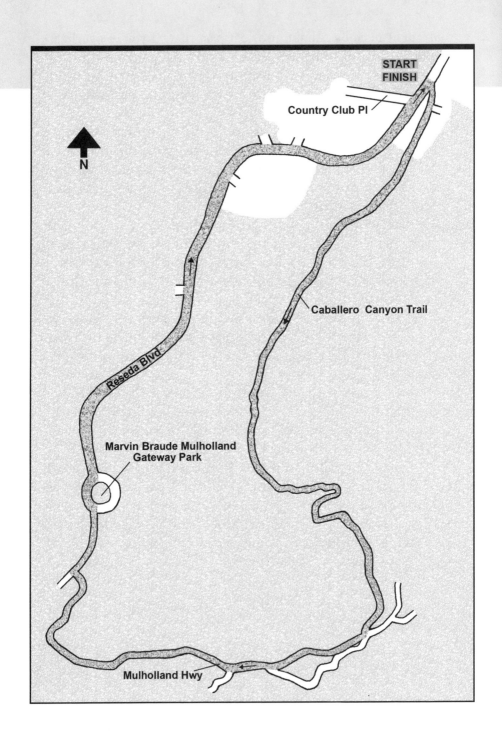

START
FINISH
Country Club Pl
N
Caballero Canyon Trail
Reseda Blvd
Marvin Braude Mulholland
Gateway Park
Mulholland Hwy

WALK #29

MULHOLLAND MARCH
DISTANCE: **4 miles**
DURATION: **2 hours**
DIFFICULTY: **3**
DETAILS: **Dogs on leash welcome. Okay for mountain bikes. Abundant free street parking. Nearest bus lines are #150, #154, #240, and #750.**

Getting out of the city and into the hills doesn't require a long drive. Sometimes, it's a short drive and a short walk. Such is the case with this hike above the Encino hills. It climbs a bit, enjoys a stretch of flat fire road, and offers tremendous views of the Valley and the beach.

Begin this walk by driving (or walking, if you're taking the bus) south on Reseda Boulevard. Go as far as Country Club Place, and park. Cross the road and look for a broad brown sign reading "Caballero Canyon." Look for a trail just to the right of this sign, and drop down into the aforementioned canyon.

Walk south (or uphill) along the flat, sandy Caballero Canyon Trail as it winds through low-growing scrub and brush. For now, ignore the little trails that come in from your right. Instead, carry on straight ahead. When you've walked 15 or 20 minutes, the trail will jog to the left and begin to rise.

Follow this main trail, again ignoring multiple narrower trail options that appear, and continue climbing. It's a bit of a workout, but trust me, it will all be worth it in a little while.

Finally the trail will finish climbing, flatten out, and come to a wide T-intersection. This is Mulholland Highway—well, the unpaved, no automobile traffic part of it, anyway.

Once long ago, it was possible to take this motorway from Hollywood all the way to the ocean. The road began near the top of Beachwood Canyon (where Lake Hollywood is now) and ran through Hollywood, across what is now the Hollywood Freeway, across what is now the San Diego Freeway, and all the way across the ridgeline you're standing on. It ended near the Los Angeles-Ventura County Line, and could be driven the whole way.

Now, of course, you can still drive from the Hollywood Sign to just west of the San Diego Freeway, and again from Topanga Canyon out to Malibu Canyon, and out to Kanan Dume Road, and all the way to the sea.

The dirt part you're on now, however—that's for walkers, hikers, bikers, and equestrians.

Turn right onto Mulholland, and begin walking as it heads west. Follow the road as it rises and falls, enjoying big views of Encino and the Sepulveda Basin off to your right. You will probably be able to see Lake Balboa from here, the nearby Japanese Garden, and a smattering of golf courses. If it's clear out, you may see all the way to Pacoima and the mountains beyond.

To your left, through cuts in the hills (or from any of the small peaks, if you want to climb a bit more), you'll find views of West Los Angeles, the Getty Center, Westwood, Santa Monica, the ocean, and the coastline south to Palos Verdes. If it's clear out, you can watch airplanes take off and land at LAX.

After about three miles of walking along Mulholland, you'll come to a flat spot that supports a white wooden signboard. Take the trail here and begin to descend. In a few minutes, you'll find yourself walking through the pay parking lot for Marvin Braude Mulholland Gateway Park. This is part of the legacy of the late city councilman who loved these mountains and was tireless in his efforts to protect them from development.

You'll find public restrooms and drinking fountains here, as well as a variety of placards bearing information about the area's geography, flora, and fauna.

Take the trail to the right of the road (or stay on the asphalt) and walk slowly downhill. After fifteen minutes or so, you'll come to the signpost for Caballero Canyon, and you'll be back where you started.

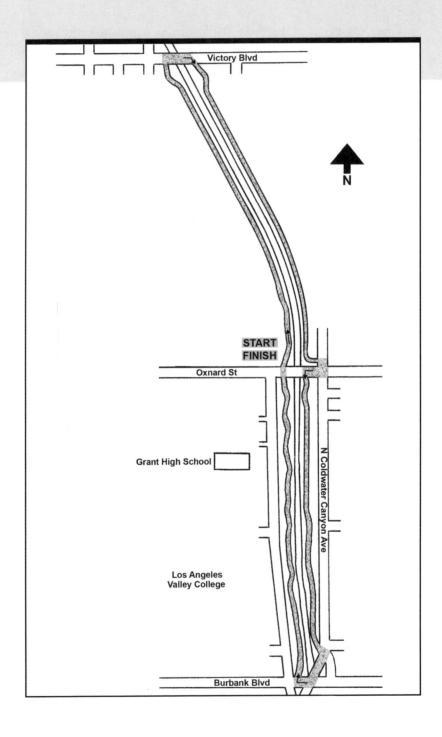

WALK #30

TUJUNGA WASH ART WALK
DISTANCE: **2.5 miles**
DIFFICULTY: **1**
DURATION: **1 hour**
DETAILS: **Ample street parking.**
Dogs on leash allowed.
Wheelchair accessible.
Metro buses #154 and #167.

This walk, while grittier and less bucolic than others, is a combination leg stretch, history lesson, and art gallery.

Begin this stroll on the northwest corner of Coldwater Canyon Avenue and Oxnard Street. Head west on Oxnard and turn right into the pathway on the west side of the wash. Pass through a set of artful green gates adorned with images of marsh plants and water birds and begin walking down the paved pathway, going north along the concrete wash.

The wash itself channels floodwater from Hansen Dam, nine miles to the north, where it collects run-off from Big Tujunga Creek and Little Tujunga Creek. Ultimately, it contributes its waters to the Los Angeles River. It's wide and deep and, most of the time, bone dry.

The garden along its western edge is a dry example of Southern California landscape, dotted with natives like the California sycamore, cactus, and sage, and non-natives like the eucalyptus.

The concrete walkway gives out very quickly and becomes a graveled path. Off to the left is a dry, narrow arroyo with a rocky streambed. When water is flowing in the wash, some of it gets diverted into this little stream, which runs for almost a mile. Follow this past a green bench, averting your eyes from the backsides of the stucco apartment buildings on the other side of the channel.

When you arrive at Victory Boulevard, if you like, you may continue walking up the wash by crossing Victory at the stoplight, jogging slightly left, and picking up the trail on the opposite side. It goes quite a distance north from here.

For this walk, though, turn right onto the sidewalk at Victory, walk fifty feet, and then turn right again to enter the walkway on the eastern side of the wash, through another set of attractive iron gates.

As you head south, you'll find that the greenery changes somewhat. Here are palo verde, oleander, lantana, and bottlebrush. Although the pathway is wider, the view is no better, and you get a closer look at the backs of those apartment buildings.

Near Oxnard, pass through a stone gate with more iron ornamentation and follow the dusty path as it enters a small green park, where older sycamores tower over a stretch of lawn. Walk to the corner and cross Oxnard Street to the lower section of Tujunga Wash.

This is where the "art gallery" begins. A public project that ran from 1976 to 1983 (with substantial restoration completed in 2011) fills the eastern-facing wall of the wash with glorious murals. This, a sign in the wash proclaims, is the "Great Wall of Los Angeles."

Taking the entire history of Los Angeles as their theme, local artists used this massive concrete canvas to create the longest mural in L.A., in work reminiscent of Diego Rivera and the muralists of the WPA.

As you walk along under some welcome, pine-scented shade, scenes from the mural include Olympic athletes of color, highlights of the civil rights and gay rights movements, the Baby Boomers and the Bracero migrant worker program, the Zoot Suit Riots, the Japanese internment camp at Manzanar, and Prohibition. Going backward in time (if you're walking south), you'll see Rosie the Riveter, the pioneers of the motion picture industry, Chinese workers building the railroads, the settlements of the Californios, the expeditions of Gaspar de Portola and Junipero Serra, and Native American Chumash villages.

It's a California history lesson in six-tenths of a mile.

At Burbank Boulevard, turn right onto the sidewalk, cross the wash, and pick up the trail on the opposite side, heading north.

You're now on the campus of Los Angeles Valley College, under more varied greenery. Here are eucalyptus and pine, as well as some flowering mulberry trees. To your left are the athletic fields of the college, a baseball diamond, an archery range, and a football stadium. In time, you will meet the bungalows of Grant High School, which shares some of this acreage with the college.

When you reach the end of the campus, you have met Oxnard Street once more—and the end of your walk.

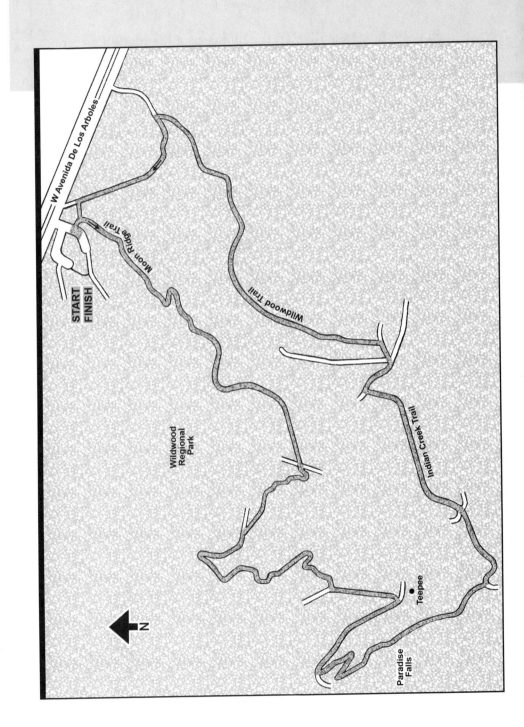

WALK #31

PARADISE FALLS
DISTANCE: **3 miles**
DURATION: **1 hour 45 minutes**
DIFFICULTY: **4**
DETAILS: **Free parking.**
Dogs on leash allowed.

This exhilarating walk is far afield for most Angelenos, but the hike and waterfall make it worth the drive. Be sure to bring water and wear good shoes. This walk has some elevation changes and includes some sections of narrow trail that will make fools of your flip-flops.

Begin this walk in Thousand Oaks, off the Ventura Freeway's (SR 134) Lynn Road exit, near the intersection of Lynn Road and Avenida De Los Arboles, at Wildwood Regional Park. You'll find plenty of street parking and a dirt parking lot, which sometimes features a portable public toilet. (You will also find more permanent public toilets back at the corner of Avenida De Los Arboles and Canna Street—one set next to the baseball fields and one next to the elementary school.)

Walk to the downhill side of the parking lot, and look for a trailhead and a set of wooden stairs. Walk down the stairs a short flight, then turn right onto the trail marked "Moonridge Trail Paradise Falls." (For now, don't take the one marked "Mesa Trail.")

This is the warm-up part of the walk. The trail will meander along, hugging the hillside and rising and falling as it passes through fields of cactus and small groves of low-growing oak. It doesn't seem a likely place for a waterfall, but as you go along you will catch glimpses of the canyon below—and of the band of greenery there, which in Southern California canyons is usually a sign of some kind of waterway.

In time, the trail will drop into a gully. Use the wooden bridge to cross the (usually) dry creek bed. When it emerges into full sun again, climb a little until you meet a wide road—Mesa Trail.

Cross the road, and continue on the narrow Moonridge Trail. It will bend right and hug the hillside before coming to some sets of wooden steps. Use these to drop down into another dry gully and then climb back out again.

Stay on the trail until it T-bones into a much wider dirt track. Turn left onto this wider road and walk down a slightly steeper grade, headed for what appears to be a large, incongruous tee-pee. This will bring some welcome shade if it's a hot day, and offer you a drinking fountain to replenish your fluids.

After you've enjoyed that, walk back uphill a short distance, the way you came to get to the teepee. Then bear left, following a wide dirt road as it heads downhill.

After about five minutes of downward grade, you'll find signs on your left for Paradise Falls. Leave the wide dirt road for a narrower trail, which can be a little slippery at times. This will drop downward via a series of switchbacks and a few sets of wooden stairs, to the canyon known as Arroyo Conejo—"Rabbit Canyon."

There, before you, will be the forty-foot cascade known as Paradise Falls.

If this seems like an unnatural place for a waterfall, well, it is. The water flowing here is headed to a water treatment facility a mile or so downstream. But it makes a delightful spot to sit and rest a bit before beginning the return journey. It's also a tempting place for a picnic, though you may want to wait until you make your way to the picnic tables a few minutes upstream.

Leaving the waterfall, climb back up the trail you descended. Halfway up, look for a trail spurring off to the right, marked

"Wildwood Trail." Follow this as it climbs along a chain-link fence, hugging the rock face closely, past the top of Paradise Falls and along the stream that feeds it. As the stream flattens, you'll see varieties of water fowl and a shaded area with several picnic tables.

Continue upstream. The trail will follow the water and then present you with a wooden bridge to cross to the other side. Once across, turn left onto Indian Creek Trail.

This path will wander along the creek, which never seems to have enough water in it to actually feed that beautiful waterfall. Here the trail will be mostly shaded, but after a time it will cross the creek again and give you a side trail option to visit Indian Cave—a shallow natural opening in the canyon wall that can be accessed via a wooden staircase.

Continue to follow the shaded creek along Wildwood Trail as it meanders back into the canyon. Eventually, staying to the left of the waterway, you will pass another small waterfall (which you will hear more clearly than you will see it) in the gully below you. Begin to climb the canyon wall, employing some switch-backs and some more wooden stair steps to gain elevation.

The trail will finally find flat ground again. Follow it across a field, from which you can see Avenida De Los Arboles off to your right. Drop down into a little shaded gully and, after a bend to the left, you will find yourself back at the wooden staircase you descended at the start of the walk.

The staircase will take you back up to the parking lot, and your starting point.

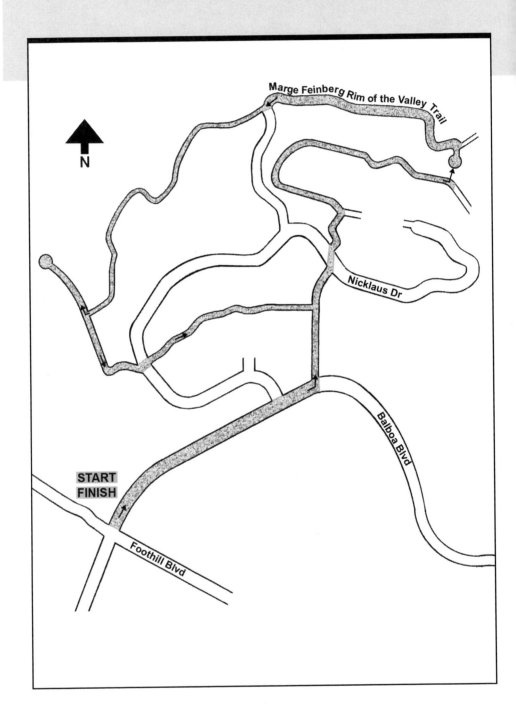

WALK #32

RIM OF THE VALLEY & L.A. AQUEDUCT
DISTANCE: **2.1 miles**
DURATION: **1 hour**
DIFFICULTY: **2**
DETAILS: **Ample street parking.**
Dogs on leash allowed.
Metro buses #236 and #237.

The construction of the Los Angeles Aqueduct turned a desert into a city and gave rise to the massive growth of the South-land in the early twentieth century. A hundred years later, the cascade of water falling into the San Fernando Valley is still a sight to behold. This walk is one of the few ways to get close enough to see it.

Begin this walk in Sylmar, near the northern end of the San Fernando Valley, at the corner of Foothill Boulevard and Balboa Boulevard. They cross in two places; this is the northern of the two crossings, very near the Golden State Freeway (I-5). Walk uphill on Balboa, heading east following a white rail fence on the left-hand side of the road.

On that same side, you can't miss the overbuilt gate for the condominium complex Legends at Cascades, at Nicklaus Drive. Walk past this for now, and continue to the crest of the hill, where you'll see a paved driveway on the left. Turn in here, and walk around the steel gate blocking auto traffic.

Follow this uphill until it crests and meets a wider paved track. Pause for a moment to take in the view.

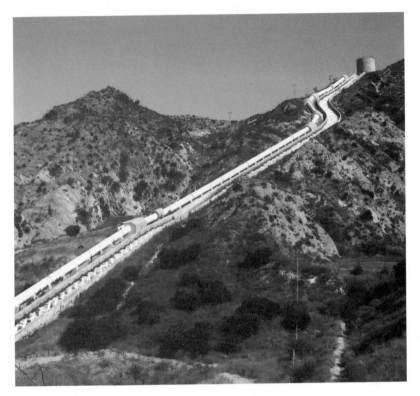

The Los Angeles Aqueduct.

The bowl and open fields that lay before you are what remain of a planned golf community, which was to include a course designed by golf legend Jack Nicklaus (hence the name of the road and the complex you just passed). Although construction did begin—far down to the right, you may be able to see a club-house—the golf course is still a dream today.

Turn left onto the paved road and walk a short distance, only twenty feet or so, to pick up a narrow concrete path on your right that winds down into the bowl. This will meet a T-intersection in a hundred feet or so. Turn left at that intersection and begin walking uphill and clockwise around the wide field.

The trail will climb and circle around to the right, passing a line of thin, forgotten pine trees. From here, you can get a better look at the remains of the Nicklaus course. Follow this path downward toward a (usually dry) pond on the right, where it will then begin to bend to the right.

As it does so, leave the path and walk to the left across open ground to the cul-de-sac end of a similar concrete path. Turn left and walk uphill, paralleling the path you've just descended.

Near the crest, this path will merge with a paved road—part of an extended trail along the foothills known as the Marge Feinberg Rim of the Valley Trail, named after a hiking enthusiast who was instrumental in keeping some of this land open for walking.

Walk straight ahead a short distance on this wide road, passing an overgrown path doubling back to the right, and then veer slightly right onto another narrow concrete pathway.

Watch for wildlife, too—I've seen deer, coyotes, and red-tailed hawks here—as the path winds its way downhill and grows gradually steeper.

The path will bottom out and hit another T-intersection. Turn right and walk a short distance to the end. Here you can get a pretty good view of the Los Angeles Aqueduct—unless it's another drought year—as it pumps its precious water into the thirsty city from hundreds of miles north in the Owens Valley.

Turn around and return the way you came—but at the T-intersection, don't turn left and go back uphill. Instead, walk straight on, as the path runs into the back of the Legends at Cascades complex.

The concrete path will meet a paved road (Nicklaus Drive) and continue on the other side. Follow it as it threads between the Legends buildings, climbing up and bending around to the right, and then circling the edge of an open field.

When you hit paved road, turn right and walk past the steel gate you passed on your way in. Then turn right again on Balboa Boulevard and walk downhill past the Legends of Cascades entryway. When you come to Foothill Boulevard, you will be back at your starting point.

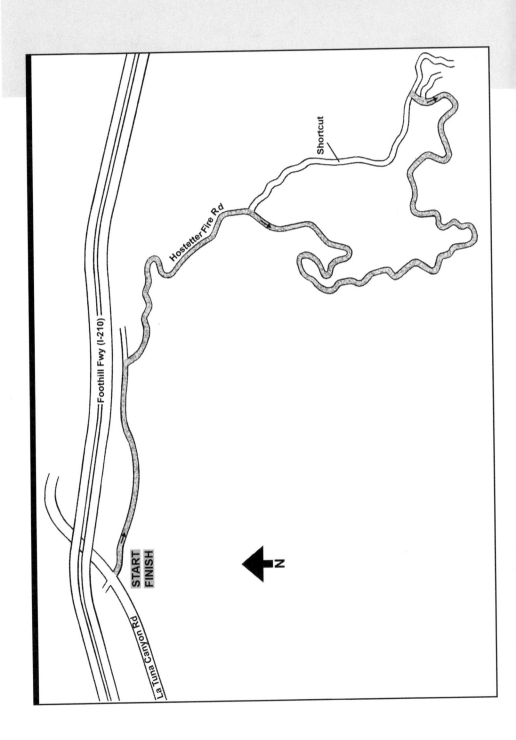

WALK #33

LA TUNA CANYON
DISTANCE: **5 miles**
(3.9 miles for the tougher version)
DURATION: **2 hours 30 minutes**
(2 hours for the tougher version)
DIFFICULTY: **3 (5 for the tougher version)**
DETAILS: **Free parking.**
Dogs on leash allowed.
No facilities at trailhead.

This is more of a workout than a walk, a steady climb into the hills punctuated by the offer of a sudden steep incline. The trail offers virtually no shade. Climb early in the day, or on a cool day, and bring plenty of water. Bring sturdy shoes with good soles—and strong legs, if you want to do the tougher version.

This walk is like an interrogation scene in a bad movie: we can do this the easy way, or we can do this the hard way. There is a shortcut, in other words, that turns this walk into a tough hike—not that the easy way is all that easy. Either way, this is a workout.

Begin from the parking area just off the Foothill Freeway (I-210), south of the freeway, at La Tuna Canyon Road. Start by walking up a slight grade on cracked asphalt with a faded yellow stripe down the middle.

Walk along the oaky hillside dotted with wildflowers, Spanish Broom, and an occasional patch of cactus. (*La tuna* is the

Spanish word for "cactus," but there isn't much of it growing
here.) The path will gradually begin to offer views of the noisy
210 Freeway and the San Gabriel Mountains. A sharp-eyed
walker may spot a set of bee boxes on the other side of the highway, where hives are making honey.

After about a third of a mile, the wide pavement ends. Turn
right onto a narrower road, which in time will show you a sign
designating it as "Hostetter." Begin walking up the slightly
steeper climb.

The road will soon flatten and begin to offer nice views of
the communities of Tujunga, La Crescenta, and Montrose. Pass
a sign that warns you to "Slow," but ignore it. You can go as fast
as you like here.

When the pavement ends, the road will slope down slightly.
The freeway noise will then fade away and give over to birdsong.

At about the 0.8-mile mark, you will meet that shortcut, in
the form of a wide trail rising up on the left. A short visual in-
spection will tell you what you need to know: it's steep and slippery and made of sandstone, with lots of loose, sandy soil and
rock.

Some walkers—the ones with good shoes, good soles, and
strong legs—use this path for this portion of the walk. If you
don't care to join them, bear right and continue up the gentler
climb on the road, which rises gradually past a ravine filled with
sycamore trees, suggesting a natural spring or perhaps a seasonal creek to feed them.

The road will gradually gain elevation. Consider, as you rise,
how lucky you are not to be climbing up that shortcut.

At the 2.4-mile mark, after about an hour of walking, you
will come to the base of a small metal water tank, where the road
divides. To your left is the top of the shortcut that the more im-
petuous walkers may have taken. If you like, you can take this
same shortcut on the way back down.

Enjoy the view in front of you. Directly below, in the foreground, is the Verdugo Hills Golf Course, a swatch of cheerful
green in a mostly brown landscape. Far behind that are the San

Gabriel Mountains, with Mount Lukens in front and Mount Wilson over to the right. Between the links and the peaks are the communities of Tujunga, La Crescenta, and Montrose.

If you like, you may continue this walk even farther by bending around to the right and following the Hostetter Fire Road into the mountains. The fire road will ultimately connect to the Verdugo Motorway, which runs along the ridge of the range separating Tujunga, La Crescenta, and Montrose from Burbank and Sun Valley. Another fifteen to twenty minutes of walking will take you to a broad overlook of that area.

If not, you now have the choice to either return the way you came, making a gentle descent out of the return trip, or go wild and make your way *down* the steep shortcut.

While the latter option is not the most sensible, it can be done if you crouch low and crab-walk sideways down the hill. Be warned—you may spend some of this route inadvertently skiing down the hillside on your backside. If you stay upright, though, you will get a great quad and calf workout.

The shortcut is about 0.6 mile long, and takes about fifteen minutes to navigate. It eliminates about a mile in terms of distance, and about thirty to forty-five minutes of walking.

Whether you go short or long, follow the road straight ahead as you make your way back, walking along the unpaved portion until the pavement begins again. Turn left onto the main road when you reach it.

Head straight back down the paved portion of the road, which will give you views of the big cooling towers in Arleta/Pacoima. Descend until you are back at the parking lot, and your starting point.

PART EIGHT

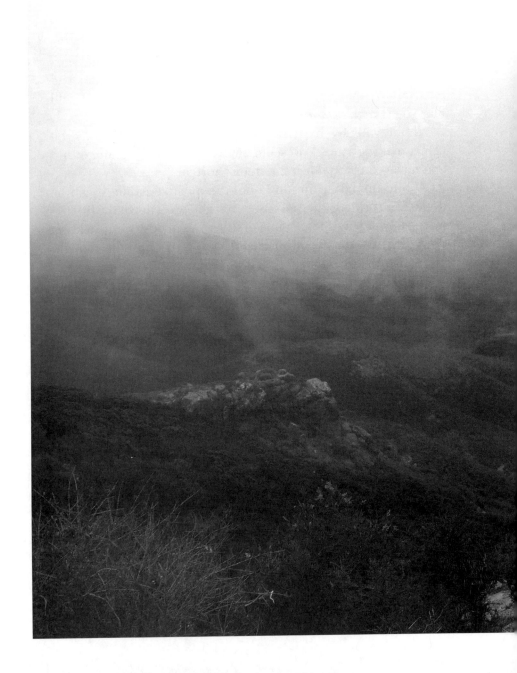

WEST
LOS ANGELES
& BEACHES

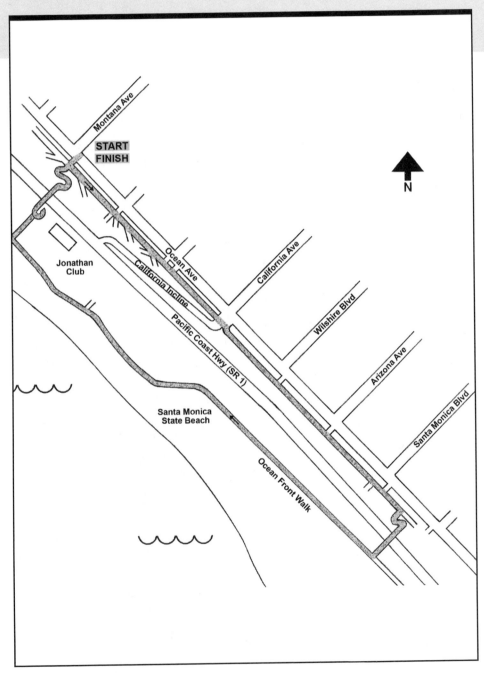

Overleaf: Along the trail near Sandstone Peak.

WALK #34

BEACH & BLUFFS WALK
DISTANCE: **3 miles**
DURATION: **1 hour 30 minutes**
DIFFICULTY: **4**
DETAILS: **Metered street parking. Dogs on leash allowed. Metro buses #20 and #534; Santa Monica buses #1 and #7.**

The bluffs and the beach below this walk make it one of Southern California's loveliest strolls, offering some of the best ocean views in Los Angeles. It is also a gambol through local history. This walk can be turned into a real workout by including some of the sets of giant steps that connect the top to the bottom.

This walk is best begun on Ocean Avenue, near its intersection with Montana Avenue, in part because it's generally easier to find parking there. Once you've parked, walk to the west side of Ocean and find the set of wooden steps going down to the beach. Use this as a landmark, and as your starting point.

Begin walking south—with the ocean, the steps, and the Pacific Coast Highway (SR 1) on your right—along a stretch of greenery known as the Santa Monica Palisades or Palisades Park. (Not to be confused with Pacific Palisades, which is the next community to the north and has its own Palisades Park, nor with the 1962 Freddy Cannon pop song of the same title, which is about an amusement park in New Jersey. The word "palisades" is a geological term that signifies a certain kind of bluff.) The area you're walking in now is actually a twenty-six-acre park along the bluffs, spread out over 1.5 miles.

On the right, you can see the historic Santa Monica Pier, with its Ferris wheel, restaurants, and ancient carousel, as well as the multimillion-dollar homes that line the oceanfront. Depending on the weather, you may be able to see Malibu on your right and Catalina Island off to your left, or even the Channel Islands in-between.

There are some equally interesting features on the path in front of you, though somewhat more hidden from view. Somewhere along here are the palm trees featured in the madcap 1963 comedy *It's a Mad, Mad, Mad, Mad World*. Also along here are the shopping cart "parking lots"—little fenced corrals where the homeless people of the area are allowed to store their belongings.

In addition to the *Mad, Mad* trees, there is a profusion of interesting tree life here. The flora includes almost a dozen types of palms, from date palms to fan palms to royal palms. You will also see the elegant Monterey cypress, varieties of pines, and several kinds of eucalyptus—said to have been planted here at the suggestion of Abbot Kinney, the developer of nearby Venice and a big proponent of the values of the Australian import. Kinney may have also encouraged the planting of the low-growing shrub, peculiar to this park, known as the Australian tea tree.

As you walk, you'll begin to see the California Incline rising up from the Pacific Coast Highway. Note the pedestrian walkway over the PCH, too, if you're interested in adding some climbing to this walk.

Staying on Ocean, continue walking south, and cross California Avenue. Across Ocean, you'll see the Fairmont Hotel. Straight ahead, across California, is a ship's mast, or maybe a ship's prow, facing the ocean. This art piece, known as Beacon Overlook, is a tribute to the military. Just beyond the overlook is a stone honoring the achievements of Juan Cabrillo, the explorer who sailed into Santa Monica Bay in 1542.

Walk close to the edge of the bluffs. From here onward, you may notice the handrails are of the "faux-bois" variety, made of concrete but shaped to look like wood—a Hollywood trick that you will see in parts of Griffith Park, too.

You may also notice that the path begins to seem a bit irregular, curving along with the contour of the bluffs. In some places, you may notice that sections of the walkway are closed. This is because the contour of the bluffs keeps changing. Periodically, a bit of the unsteady sandstone below gives way, and the walkway has to be moved inland a few feet to make it safe for walking.

At the Wilshire Boulevard intersection, stop for a moment and pay your respects to the strangely phallic statue of Saint Monica, a concrete carving from 1934. She is known principally for her forbearance of her husband's flagrant adultery. She is also the mother of Saint Augustine, he of the "Confessions."

There are also tributes along here to John P. Jones, co-founder of Santa Monica, and Arcadia Bandini de Stearns Baker, the widow of Jones's co-founder, Colonel Robert S. Baker. They donated the land for this park.

Continue south. At the next intersection, which is Arizona Avenue, note the elegant Shangri La Hotel across Ocean Avenue. On your right, you will see a set of steps. This was once the location of the "99 Steps," a huge wooden staircase that dropped down to the sand before the PCH was built.

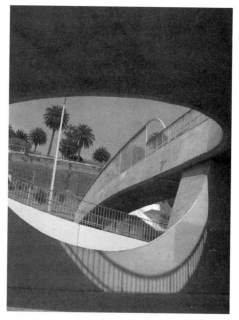

This modern stairway replaced the original wooden "99 Steps" staircase.

Today, it's a modern staircase that leads to a bridge that crosses *over* PCH and deposits you near the bike path that runs along the beach.

If you're feeling frisky, you can trot down and back up the stairs for an extra workout, or turn your walk into a figure-eight by including these stairs and coming up the ones by the California Incline. Up to you!

A little farther down, past the intersection of Ocean and Santa Monica Boulevard, make sure you don't miss the Georgian Hotel. This 1933 Art Deco construction, once an elegant private residence, is one of Santa Monica's best-preserved and most beautiful buildings.

As you continue south, you will come to a cannon, said to be from the Civil War and believed to have been placed here, facing the sea, as another tribute to John P. Jones and the widow Arcadia Bandini de Stearns Baker.

Beyond this is the famed Camera Obscura, a "darkroom" that uses the combined power of darkness inside, sunshine outside, and a lens between, to project images of the surrounding area onto a screen, like a living, breathing movie of the reality outside. Built in 1899, it is a wonder that is well worth the side trip.

Just past this is a more modern note. For decades, the city maintained a few shuffleboard courts for the use of its elderly citizens. These are now gone. In their place: bocce ball courts. A sign of the times.

Return to the cannons and look toward the bluffs. There, you'll find a staircase. Drop down a set of brick steps, leading to a curved walkway over the PCH and culminating in set of concrete steps down to ground level. Walk toward the water, and find the pedestrian and bicycle paths that run along the sand.

For a side trip, turn left and explore the Santa Monica Pier if you feel like having a snack or paying a visit to the wonderful old 1915 carousel—a relatively late addition to the pier, which was built in 1909 and once featured a 15,000-square-foot ballroom and a roller coaster known as the "Blue Streak Racer."

Otherwise, turn right and head north, with the ocean on

your left, along the sidewalk known as Ocean Front Walk.

This stretch of beach was once lined with elegant, private beach clubs. The parking lot just to your right was built on the ruins of the old Deauville Beach Club, destroyed by a fire in 1955. As you walk along, you may sense the ghosts of the Casa Del Mar, Sorrento, Edgewater, and Miramar clubs. You will also pass clubs that do still exist, such as the Jonathan Club, near the base of the California Incline, and the Beach Club, a little farther north.

Walk on, watching out for bicyclists, who have the right of way, and skaters. Where the sidewalk ends, join the bike path as it winds left across the sand. Continue until you have reached the Jonathan Club (evident from its "Members Only" signs and many umbrellas and beach chairs in the sand).

Walk into the parking lot just before the Jonathan Club and look for a circular staircase that looks like a snail shell. (Look for the public restrooms here, too, if you need those.) Head for the staircase, but before beginning the climb up, notice something odd. In the sidewalk, along the edge of the PCH, you can see tiles that spell out "The Gables."

Across the highway, embedded in the sandstone, you will see the remains of a structure formerly known as the Gables, which was perhaps the most ambitious hotel in this beach community. Built in the 1920s, the Gables was originally planned to include twenty stories of rooms and suites, rising up to and above the level of Palisades Park and spreading out across the PCH below with beachfront suites. In reality, the Gables only rose three stories before time and the Depression got the better of it. What you see now is all that remains.

Wind your way around the snail shell staircase, up and across the PCH, and then begin the stair climb that will take you back to the park. The top of the staircase lands near Montana Avenue. You are back at your starting point.

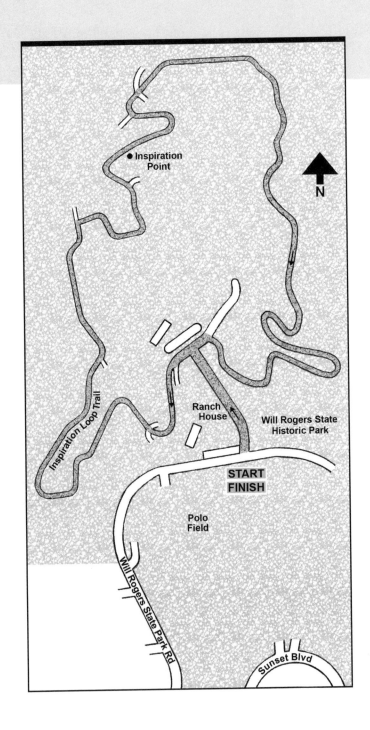

Inspiration Point

N

Inspiration Loop Trail

Ranch
House

Will Rogers State
Historic Park

START
FINISH

Polo
Field

Will Rogers State Park Rd

Sunset Blvd

WALK #35

WILL ROGERS STATE HISTORIC PARK
DISTANCE: **2.5 miles**
DURATION: **1 hour**
DIFFICULTY: **2**
DETAILS: **Free street parking;**
$12 paid parking.
Dogs on leashes allowed.
Metro buses #2 and #302.

This is a pleasant, undemanding hike from one of Los Angeles's most beautiful historic homes up into hills that offer some of the city's most captivating coastal views. It's also one of the city's best picnic spots. If you go on the right weekend, you can even catch a free polo match.

Begin your walk at the gates of the old Will Rogers estate, accessed from Sunset Boulevard, off of Will Rogers State Park Road and east of Chautauqua Boulevard. Park on the streets outside the park grounds, or pay to park inside.

Walk up to the house itself, a low-lying ranch-style home where the great cowboy, actor, writer, and political commentator made his home from 1920 to 1935. Rogers was a very popular figure in his time. Born in Oklahoma's Cherokee territory, the droll midwesterner was a cowboy who went on to develop a circus act (which turned into a rope and pony act on Vaudeville), work in both silent movies and talkies, write syndicated columns for the *New York Times* and the *Saturday Evening Post*, and host a nationally syndicated radio show.

Before he died in a plane crash while traveling in Alaska with aviator Wiley Post in 1935, Rogers had become Hollywood's highest-paid actor and one of the nation's most prominent progressive voices. Some of his most famous quotes are: "I am not a member of an organized political party; I am a Democrat," "Diplomacy is the art of saying 'nice doggie' until you can find a rock," and "I never met a man I didn't like." (During the sixties, liberal pundits

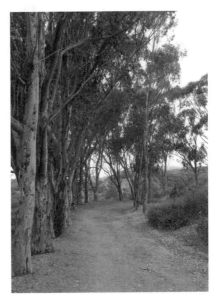

A corridor of eucalyptus trees on the trail.

liked to quote this last line and point out that Rogers never met Richard Nixon.)

Many years after Rogers's death, his widow, Betty, deeded the ranch, buildings, and grounds of the estate to the state of California, on the condition that polo be played there. So, below the house is a polo field where, on Saturday and Sunday afternoons from April to October, members of the Will Rogers Polo Club come to ride and play. I spent many a Sunday afternoon here, picnicking, in my younger years.

Above the house are stables where the polo ponies are kept. Horses are also available there for guided trail ride rentals. The home itself is open for tours Thursday through Sunday.

Begin your walk on the paved service road between the house and the stables going uphill from the main parking lot, between a wide green lawn and a group of picnic tables. Take this road until it meets the stables and a riding ring. To the right is a display of Will Rogers-era blacksmithery; to the left is the base of Inspiration Loop Trail.

Begin walking the trail, noting as you go that it is a shared path. You may expect to meet some other hikers, and perhaps some folks on horseback, too.

The first mile of this walk is a gentle climb, much of it shaded by rows of eucalyptus and studded with oak, sumac, and bay laurel trees. The elevation gain is gradual—you'll hardly know that you're climbing. But the improving views to the west will suggest otherwise, as the Pacific Ocean and some of the beaches slowly reveal themselves.

After one mile, where you will find a signpost for Inspiration Point, turn right onto a narrow dirt path. A few minutes later, take a left onto a similarly narrow trail that climbs a hill via a set of railroad tie stairs, to the top of Inspiration Point.

(If you miss this, don't worry. In time, the main trail will curve around and give you another way to get to the little peak.)

Here the view is spectacular—you can see the ocean, the beaches, Santa Monica and its pier, the South Bay, and more. The benches and tables make it easy to enjoy the view with a rest stop or a picnic.

Descend from Inspiration Point on the opposite side from where you made the climb up, dropping back down to the loop trail and turning right.

In time, you'll come to the entrance for Backbone Trail. One of Southern California's principal hiking destinations, this trail begins here and continues for an unbroken fifty-five miles to the north, winding through Topanga and Malibu Canyons and finally ending at Point Mugu, near Oxnard.

Pass the trail entrance and keep descending, staying on the main trail, which will lead you into a picturesque alley of old eucalyptus trees, probably planted here during Will Rogers's lifetime. You'll eventually start to catch glimpses of the park below you.

When you meet the stables, turn left onto the paved road where you started. Now, having earned it, you can enjoy that picnic and polo match.

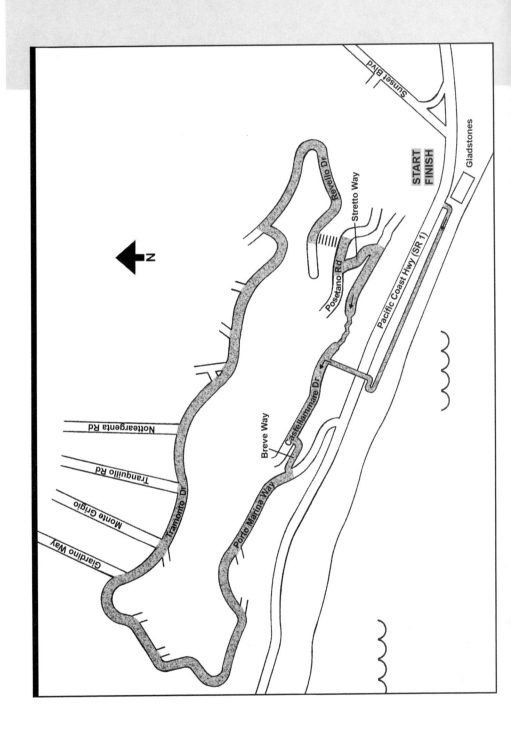

WALK #36

CASTELLAMMARE LOOP
DISTANCE: **2.6 miles**
DURATION: **1 hour 15 minutes**
DIFFICULTY: **3**
DETAILS: **Free street parking; paid lot parking. Dogs on leashes allowed. Metro buses #2, #302, and #534.**

This is a gorgeous seaside walk that takes in a stretch of coastline and some of Santa Monica's most scenic residential streets, lined with fascinating historical homes.

Locate the intersection of Sunset Boulevard and Pacific Coast Highway (SR 1), and make your way to the parking lot in front of the popular seafood restaurant Gladstones.

If you have brought a picnic lunch, you may enjoy a coastal anomaly: though Gladstones is a private establishment—owned by former Los Angeles mayor Richard Riordan—its patio and restrooms are open, for free, to the public, because the restaurant sits on public beachfront land.

So, you may approach the host or hostess and ask for a table on the patio for your picnic, or use the facilities, with happy impunity. Or you can just enjoy a Gladstones meal and enjoy the view.

Begin your walk by heading north, walking along the Gladstones property into the long, thin public parking lot just above it. Stroll along this until you come to stairs rising to a high pedestrian walkway that crosses over the PCH. Use this to get to the other side.

Raymond Chandler noted this structure in his masterwork, *Farewell, My Lovely*, published in 1940. In that novel, Chandler has his detective Philip Marlowe drive north on the PCH and park in front of a popular cafe before using the public staircase to climb high into the hills. At one point, Marlowe thinks to himself, "It was a nice walk, if you like grunting."

In Chandler's day, the large white Spanish building you're approaching on your left *was* a cafe—Thelma Todd's Sidewalk Cafe, owned by film actress Thelma Todd, who appeared in two Marx Brothers movies: *Horse Feathers* and *Monkey Business*. Todd died under mysterious circumstances, found unconscious in the front seat of her Lincoln Phaeton, a victim of carbon monoxide poisoning. Suspects in the unsolved murder included her boyfriend, her ex-husband, and the gangster Lucky Luciano, whom she was said to be dating.

The bleached-white former cafe building is now the home of the faith-based film company Paulist Productions. Admire this as you cross the PCH and walk up the short staircase on the other side. When you reach the top, take a left and begin walking on Castellammare Drive, noting as you go the public staircase on your right. You will see many of these on this walk, and could make an entire hike out of them. But that's another book, isn't it?

Already, you have fine, low-altitude ocean views, and they will only get better as you walk along. Go a block's length or so before bending left and slightly downhill on Breve Way, then bear right and slightly uphill on Porto Marina Way.

Obviously, there's a little Italian influence here. The original designers named the streets in this area after locations on the Amalfi Coast.

There is also evidence here of Mother Nature's indifference to man-made structures. This area is subject to landslides. You will see streets with buckles in the pavement, some remnants of houses that once stood here, and even more remnants of streets that no longer exist and the bits of staircases that used to connect them. The area was particularly hard hit in the 1971 Sylmar earthquake, a 6.4 temblor that killed sixty-five people.

Walk on, up Porto Marina. In time the street will bend to the right, and in its elbow is one of the city's great houses. This is Villa de Leon, named after Leon Kauffman, the wool magnate who commissioned this 1928 construction. Recently listed at $14.5 million, the 12,000-square-foot home features a circular, ocean-view dining room, a marble staircase, nine bedrooms, eleven bathrooms, a seven-car garage, and magnificent vistas from almost every room. I particularly like the wood nymphs adorning the outside gates, and the carved ram positioned over the door.

Walk on and continue gaining elevation as you pass a few more marvelous old homes. You'll soon find yourself in the newer section of Castellammare, which, like the nearby Pacific Palisades, underwent a construction boom in the 1960s. Staying to the left, you'll pass a couple of streets before Porto Marina Way turns into Tramonto Drive. This street will rise and then flatten out, providing canyon views to the left of the famed Getty Villa.

Climb on. The houses are newer here at the crest, but no less grand, and the streets are still Italian. On the left, you'll pass Vicino, Giardino, Monte Grigio, Tranquillo, Notteargenta, and more.

On the right, you'll get some of the best coastal views Los Angeles has to offer, from Point Dume down through Malibu to the Palisades, Santa Monica, and beyond. Catalina Island is often visible from here, and sometimes the Channel Islands are, too.

Also visible is more wreckage from the Sylmar earthquake. The road you're on rises and falls a bit, in a way that it didn't when it was first laid out. Below, you can see the foundations of houses that slid down the hill or were crushed by earth sliding down the hill. The asphalt here often looks new, because the hillside is still moving, and the road cracks regularly enough to need constant maintenance.

Walk on. Tramonto will come to a T-intersection. Turn right onto Revello Drive. This will begin to lower your elevation, gradually dropping downward and winding around.

This street, thanks to more earthquake destruction, narrows

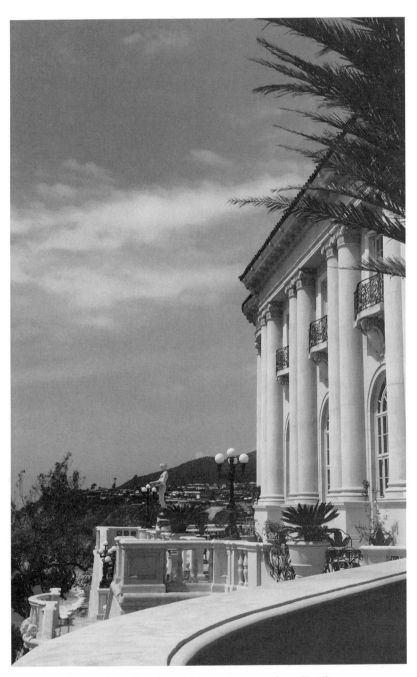

Villa de Leon, built in 1928 for wool magnate Leon Kauffman.

down to a single lane and then ends in a cul-de-sac. (Ignore the "Do Not Enter" sign, if you see one. This is meant for cars.) Just before it does, look to the left and find the short but steep public staircase that drops down one block to Posetano Road. Turn right, walk a short block, and stop at the corner of Stretto Way.

The big house with blue trim on your right is Castillo Del Mar, the house where poor Thelma Todd was living when she died. The home has been nicely preserved, and looks much as it did in her time.

Turn left on Stretto and walk downhill a block, then turn right onto Castellammare Drive once more. Here again are lovely beach views, and a few lovely old homes. (And more earthquake wreckage. Down the hill is the remnant of a walkway that used to parallel the road, a few yards above the coast highway. Now most of it is gone.)

Castellammare Drive used to continue and connect to the area you walked at the beginning of this hike. Now it ends in a cul-de-sac, but continues in a charming canyon trail. It doesn't last long—not even a hundred yards—but it is a nice break from the pavement.

On the other side, walk a short distance until you find, on your left, the staircase leading to the pedestrian walkway crossing the PCH. Use this to get to the beach side of the street, and turn left into the parking lot along the highway. Walk straight on, back to Gladstones and your starting point.

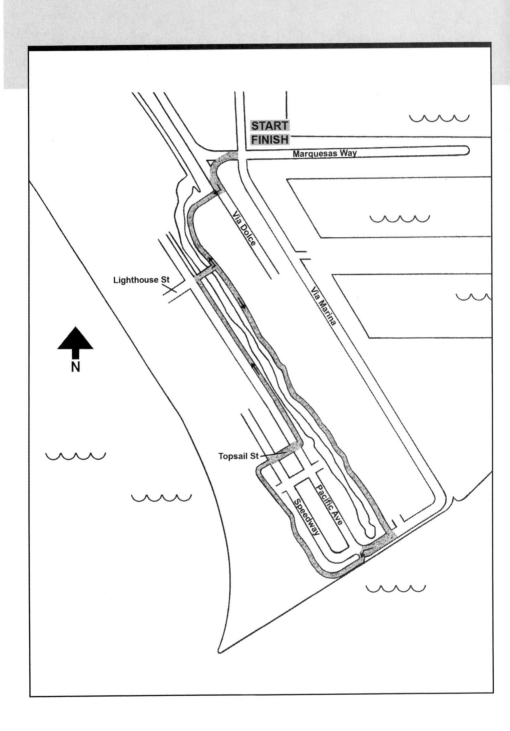

WALK #37

MARINA DEL REY'S BALLONA LAGOON
DISTANCE: **2.5 miles**
DIFFICULTY: **1**
DURATION: **1 hour**
DETAILS: **Free street parking. Paid parking available. Dogs on leash allowed. Culver City buses #1, #108, and #358.**

Here's a great way to explore the byways of Marina Del Rey's Ballona Lagoon, and to get a little seaside stroll, too.

Begin your walk in Marina Del Rey, near the intersection of Via Marina (known as Ocean Avenue, north of Washington Boulevard) and Marquesas Way. Park on the street, if you are lucky enough to find an open space, or in Parking Lot 12, just off Marquesas. Then walk west on Marquesas to Via Dolce, turn left, and begin walking with the lagoon on your right.

After a short block, pick up the dirt path coming in on the right, bordered by a split-rail redwood fence. Begin walking along South Esplanade East.

This pathway is a recent addition to the Marina landscape—and it's a welcome one. The path rises and falls gently, drops down and back up a couple of sets of redwood staircases, and trails along the waterway that carries the Ballona Lagoon waters out to the main channel of the Marina.

Along the way, on the left, you will be treated to the whimsical architectural stylings of the Marina, which include structures clad in everything from stucco to shingles and everything in-between. Several of the homeowners have invested in lawns—some plastic, some grass—and others have lovely flower gardens. All of these houses are lucky enough to have the same view from their backyards that you see now on your right, of the gentle Ballona water, the sea, and the shorebirds that call it home. You may see egrets, great blue herons, and more.

On your right, notice (but don't use) the pedestrian bridge that crosses the waterway and connects the Marina with the Marina Peninsula. This will be a useful landmark later on.

Like the pathway you're on, the Marina itself is also a fairly recent addition. Said to be the world's largest small-craft harbor—and the largest man-made harbor in the United States, with nineteen individual marinas and a capacity for almost 6,000 boats—this acreage was for centuries a salt marsh fed by Ballona Creek. In the early 1900s, developers sought to make something of the area. By the 1930s, plans were afoot to turn it into a commercial harbor. It had a shot at becoming Los Angeles's principal port, even, but lost out to San Pedro.

It wasn't until the 1960s that a breakwater was finally built to protect the area from sea swells, and construction began in earnest. The marina opened in 1966. It wasn't until some years afterward that the lots you're walking past were graded for homes.

Depending on the time of day, you may be treated to some closer-than-expected views of aircraft taking off from LAX, whose western-facing runways extend just a few miles south of here. You may also see large sails crossing before you—the tops of boats leaving the marina along the main channel.

When you hit Via Marina, cross the street carefully and stop to enjoy a view of the passing parade of boats. Across the channel, in the near distance, is the breakwater, with the famous Marvin Braude Bike Trail running along it. (The bike trail starts in the Pacific Palisades and runs almost all the way to Palos Verdes.) Beyond that is the community of Playa Del Rey. The clump of green right across the water is Del Rey Lagoon, the southern sister to Ballona Lagoon.

For now, turn right and follow the main channel. The roadway will veer right onto Pacific Avenue. But you should continue a bit, past a large, handsome, dark-colored Craftsman bungalow.

Past the house, you can either continue your seaside stroll and walk straight ahead out to the breakwater's end (perhaps another eighth of a mile), or head north along the narrow sidewalk and enjoy some beach time.

Here you will find volleyball courts and sunbathers as you walk past the doors of folks lucky enough to own real estate on this relatively deserted beachfront. (There is almost no public parking along this stretch of the Marina Peninsula, and very little street parking, which keeps the sand empty even at the height of the season.)

Off to the left, you'll note a fenced-in area of the beach. This is a protected area, set aside for an endangered bird known as the California least tern. Plovers reportedly nest nearby, too.

As you head north, you'll probably also have noticed another peculiarity of the Marina: all of the street names are alphabetical, and nautical. You will have already passed Windward and Voyage and Union Jack. As you continue, look for Topsail Street.

Here the sidewalk ends. Turn right and cross Speedway, then cross Pacific Avenue. Take a left onto another stretch of the walkway bordered by a split-rail redwood fence—the other side of the Esplanade, on the western edge of Ballona Lagoon.

Walk north, past Spinnaker, Reef, Quarterdeck, Privateer, Outrigger, North Star and Mast Streets. At Lighthouse, use the pedestrian bridge you noticed earlier to cross the waterway back to your original path.

Turn left onto South Esplanade East, and walk north the quarter-mile or so back to Via Dolce, and back to your starting point.

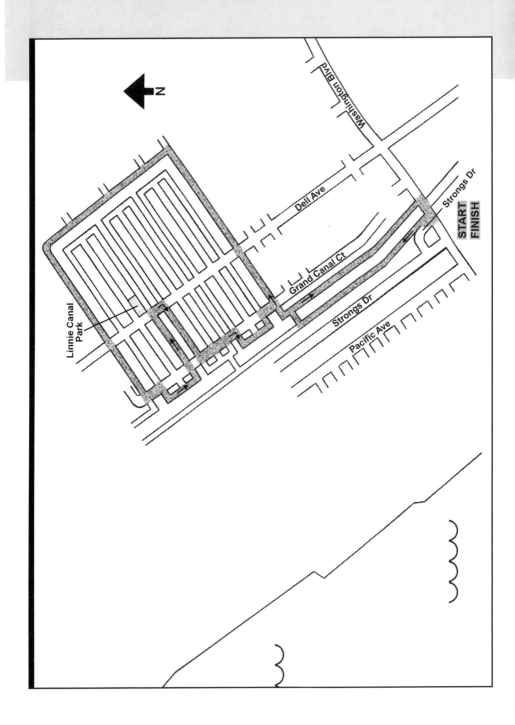

WALK #38

VENICE CANALS WALK

DISTANCE: **2 miles**
DIFFICULTY: **1**
DURATION: **1 hour 30 minutes**
DETAILS: **Free and metered street parking. Dogs on leash allowed. No bikes, boards, or blades allowed on canal walkway. Metro buses #108 and #358; Culver City bus #1.**

The imaginative real estate developer Abbott Kinney built the Venice Canals to create a West Coast artists' colony and bring prospective home buyers to the beach. Today, though only one-quarter of the original canals remain, the area is among the city's most prized neighborhoods. It's a cool spot for a walk on a hot day.

Begin this walk near the intersection of Washington Boulevard and Pacific Avenue, at the corner of Washington and Strongs Drive. Here, under a small sign that reads "Venice Canals Walkway," turn in and begin exploring.

At the turn of the last century, developer Abbott Kinney built an ambitious series of interlocking canals in a marshy district near the beach, filling the entire quadrant of Washington Boulevard to the south, Venice Boulevard to the north, Pacific Avenue to the west, and what is now Abbott Kinney Boulevard to the east.

Kinney designed the community, known as the "Venice of America," so that each home would have a canal-facing front yard. He connected the canals by a series of narrow bridges.

The area had recently been connected to the outside world by the completion of a railway line to the ocean, and an extension of Los Angeles's famed electric trolley car system. This and the new canals helped lead to the real estate development's success—especially after Kinney imported gondolas and gondoliers from Venice, Italy.

By the end of the Second World War, though, the canals were a foul mess, and the sidewalks fronting them were unsafe for walking. Much of the area was drained, and many of the canals were closed and paved over.

A huge reclamation effort, though, restored much of the former grandeur, and by the mid-1990s the Venice Canals district had once again become a prized address. Today, it is one of the richest per-square-foot real estate areas in the city.

Walk along the sidewalk on the western edge of the canal. At the first wooden pedestrian bridge you meet, turn right, cross the bridge, and turn left. Follow the sidewalk a short distance until it turns right and follows the water.

This is another world. The traffic noises are gone. The homes—which vary from monster McMansions to little bungalows that might be untouched from the original 1905 construction—are landscaped with a California cornucopia of agapanthus, day lilies, honeysuckle, bougainvillea, sage, and lavender. This being Venice, the smell of incense is often in the air.

The canals are clean and calm, with moored kayaks, canoes, and rowboats bobbing in the water. On two long morning walks here, I saw no one actually using the water on any of these watercraft, but almost every home seems to have some small seagoing vessel moored in front of it.

Continue along this sidewalk, passing another wooden pedestrian bridge and then crossing a reinforced car bridge. (This would be Dell Avenue.) When you come to the sidewalk's end, turn left and follow the water north as you walk along Eastern

Canal.

Shortly, you will pass a fence made of metal flamingos, then the bridges of Court B, Court C, and Court D. (These are car bridges, which people use to access their homes and garages on the canals.)

When you get to the end of the sidewalk, which also marks the end of the Eastern Canal, turn left once again. Note the "castle" across the water, right next to a large Moorish-Italianate home and two over from a Craftsman on steroids. That's Southern California architecture for you!

Walk on, eventually crossing Dell Avenue again and continuing until you reach the next pedestrian bridge, on your left. Cross this, then turn right on the other side and walk along the canal until you reach the sidewalk's end. Turn left, walk to the next corner, and turn left again.

You are now on Linnie Canal walk. Go past a pedestrian bridge on your right and continue until you meet Dell Avenue again. Across the street, you will see a quaint little park with play structures for the children and a small pond for the ducks. (If you're with a dog, these are both off-limits.)

Turn right onto Dell, cross the canal, and turn right again, walking west along another length of quiet canal. Continue to the end of the sidewalk, turn left, and follow the canal south. Turn left at the next corner, where the sidewalk ends again, then take the next pedestrian bridge over the water. Turn left and follow the sidewalk along the canal again.

You'll follow this same maneuver once more—getting to the sidewalk's end, turning left, crossing a pedestrian bridge, and turning right—until you have crossed the last of Venice's little islands. (You'll know you're there because you'll pass the first pedestrian bridge that you crossed at the beginning of this walk.)

Follow this last sidewalk along the canal, until it takes you back to Washington Boulevard and your starting point.

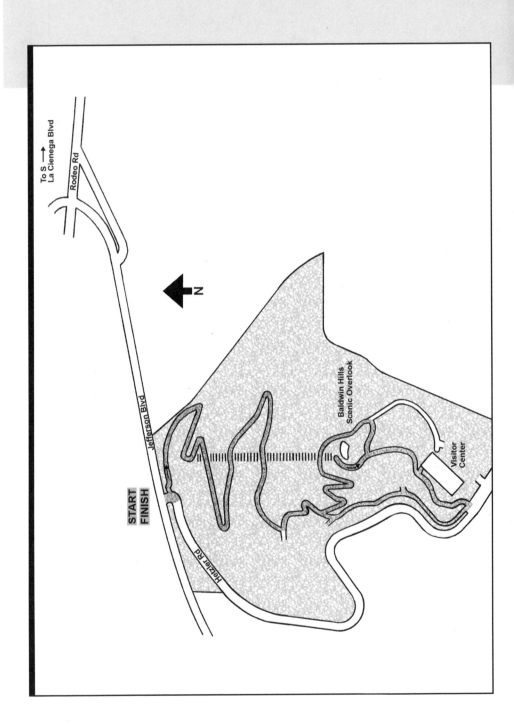

START
FINISH

To S →
La Cienega Blvd

Rodeo Rd

Jefferson Blvd

N

Hetzler Rd

Baldwin Hills
Scenic Overlook

Visitor
Center

WALK #39

BALDWIN HILLS SCENIC OVERLOOK
DISTANCE: **2.5 miles**
DURATION: **1 hour**
DIFFICULTY: **3 (or 5)**
DETAILS: **Free street parking.**
Park closed from sunset
to 8 am. No dogs allowed.
Culver City bus #4.

Culver City isn't known for its scenic views or hiking trails. But this relatively new city park offers both—a gentle walk up to an elevation that offers an unexpected perspective on the skyline stretching from Westwood to downtown L.A. It also offers a steep, heart-stopping staircase for those interested in a real workout.

Begin this walk at the base of Baldwin Hills, west of the intersection of Rodeo Road and South La Cienega Boulevard, where Jefferson Boulevard meets Hetzler Road. Park on the street—or drive up Hetzler for $6 paid parking (and handicapped parking) at the top of the hill, by the visitor center. (Note that this lot is unattended, and the parking may require exact change.)

Enter the park from Jefferson, past a sign that reads "Baldwin Hills Scenic Overlook." Follow the path marked "Trailhead" and begin walking uphill. This will take you through a few wide, slow switchbacks as you gently gain a little elevation.

Then . . . the stairs.

This park is most famous for its stairs—a set of 282 massive

stone steps, unevenly spaced and very tall, that look from a distance like a miniature Great Wall of China. They are very popular with the extreme exercise crowd.

You may see some of these folks *running* up the stairs. You
may see some of them running while wearing ankle weights or
those vests filled with water, designed to make a mockery of
anyone who's just plain hiking.

If you want to join them, please do. The stairs cross the path
several times on the ascent. You can take them part of the way or
all the way to the top, where the path and the stairs meet.

Otherwise, continue walking up the dirt path, enjoying on
each switchback a slightly improved view of the city spreading
out behind you.

The land you're walking on was once the location of an oil
field, with a drinking water reservoir at the top. The city purchased the land in 2000, and spent the next nine years removing
what was not native to the site, adding back what was, and creat-
ing a staircase out of the blocks of concrete that were left here.

The fifty-seven-acre park is home to a variety of snakes,
small mammals, and birds, and supports a habitat of common
native plants. (One morning, I surprised—and was surprised
by—a king snake that was napping on one of the big concrete
steps.) Purple and white sage grows here, and you'll see examples of the red-berried toyon plant growing low to the ground,
too.

The walk doesn't offer a lot of shade—there may not be a single tree in this park—but the increasing elevation and relative
proximity to the ocean mean there's often a cooling sea breeze
blowing in from the west.

Climb on as the trail winds upward, criss-crossing the staircase where those show-offs huff and puff their way up and down
the big steps.

In time, you will arrive at a wide concrete viewing platform
set at the top of the hill, at around 500 feet above sea level. Stop
now, and catch your breath while you catch the view.

It's an almost 360-degree panorama. From your far left you

get the ocean, Palos Verdes, Catalina Island, maybe one of the Channel Islands, and the coastline extending past Malibu to Point Dume.

In the center, you have Culver City, with the huge Sony lot (formerly MGM) just below you, and the communities of Santa Monica, West Los Angeles, Westwood, Century City, Beverly Hills, the Miracle Mile, and downtown L.A. stretching in the foreground, with the Sunset Strip, Hollywood Hills, Griffith Park Observatory, and other famous landmarks in the background.

Far to the right, you can see as far as Mount Baldy and, on a clear winter day, even the snow-capped mountains above Big Bear.

For the return, you can either retrace your steps down the curving trail, or, if your knees are up to it, walk down the big steps.

I like to break up the walk with a visit to the visitors center. To do that, leave the concrete platform headed to the left (if you're facing the city) and walk along the paved path to a low, attractive building set just off the peak of the hill. Here you will find bathrooms, drinking fountains, and informative plaques and exhibits. (The center is open from 9 AM to 4 PM, and the event space is available for weddings and parties.)

Wind through the plant garden, which will identify some of the native flora for you. Then begin walking on the road that extends down from the parking lot.

As the road leaves the lot, look for a wide dirt trail on the right. Take this, and begin angling downhill and away from the road. When you are well away from it, and you come to a fork in the road, take the left-hand option to return to the trail that brought you to the top.

Then angle down and right again, staying away from the road. Eventually you will cross the giant steps again. Continue on the trail, following the switchbacks and crossing the steps two more times as you make your way back downhill.

Eventually the trail returns you to the spot where Hetzler meets Jefferson, and to your starting point.

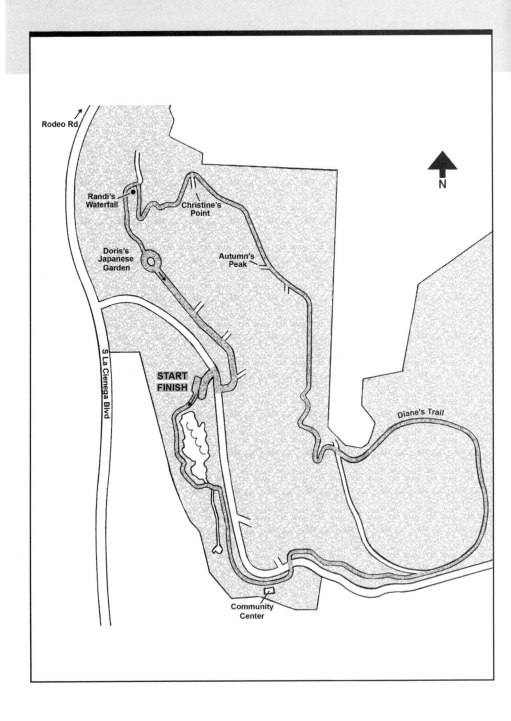

WALK #40

KENNETH HAHN STATE RECREATION AREA
DISTANCE: **2.8 miles**
DURATION: **1 hour 15 minutes**
DIFFICULTY: **2.5**
DETAILS: **Dogs on leash allowed. Lake, waterfall, and Bowl Loop areas are wheelchair accessible. Free parking except on weekends and holidays, when it's $6.**

This is a surprisingly lush walk in the unlikeliest of places— off La Cienega Boulevard, surrounded by barren hills dotted with oil-pumping equipment. But within the 308-acre park are vast lawns, groves of eucalyptus, sumac, and oaks, several small lakes, a rushing stream, and a Japanese garden. And some of the best city views in Los Angeles.

Begin this walk off La Cienega Boulevard, south of Rodeo Road, following the signs for Kenneth Hahn State Recreation Area. Exit La Cienega, follow the driveway uphill into the park, drive past the parking kiosk—or, if it's a weekend day, stop and pay your six dollars—and turn in at the first parking lot on your right.

Now you can begin walking. Head downhill past a set of public restrooms, toward a large artificial lake dotted with ducks and other water birds. (Signs, ignored by many visitors, ask you not to feed the ducks.) Curve around the right side of the lake, making a circle around the shoreline.

Kenneth Hahn was a lifelong Los Angeles politician born and raised in the central part of the city, who for forty years toiled as a county supervisor. He died in 1997, but this 400-acre park was dedicated in his name in 1984.

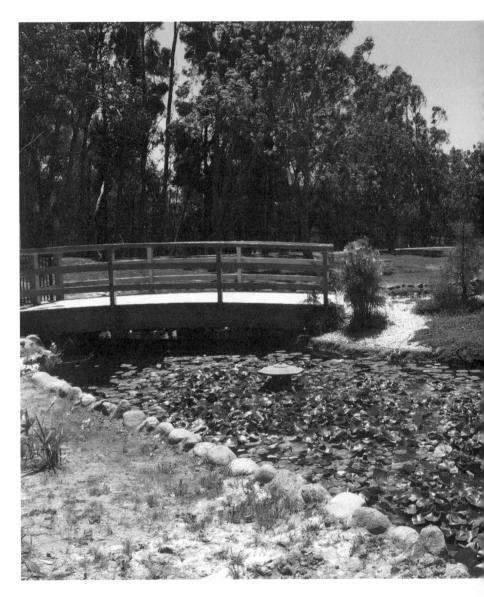

Curve around the lake, past picnic tables and BBQ grills. At the far end, cross the artificial stream that fills the lake and curve right to walk uphill along the stream bed.

As you go, look across the canyon to your right. You'll see dry, scrubby hillside, interrupted by the praying mantis-like iron structures pumping oil out of the ground.

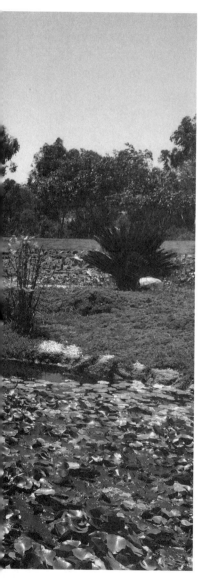

That's what this parkland looked like before it became a state recreation center. It may be a little tacky with the fake stream and lake, but consider the alternative.

Continue walking uphill, past more picnic tables, aiming for a community center building on the right where you can get a map of the park (for some reason, this is *not* available at the parking kiosk near the entrance). Walk past this, too, and continue as the path parallels a road.

Cross the road at the stop sign and use the left-hand side to walk up a steeper slope, passing a drinking fountain and a picnic table to get to the crest of the hill.

Now things get interesting. Before you is a vast green bowl—identified by one sign as Janice's Green Valley—covered in grassy lawn and decorated with oak trees. Not a natural canyon, nor a dell, this is what remains of a reservoir that once held 290 million gallons of drinking water.

In December 1963, the dam holding

The lotus-filled ponds of Doris's Japanese Garden.

that water gave way. The resulting deluge killed five people and destroyed hundreds of homes in the neighborhoods below. The collapse has historical media significance, too: it is the first natural disaster ever reported using live television and helicopter footage. The YouTube videos are impressive.

Walk straight on, keeping the bowl on your left and an exercise station on your right. Find the wide gravel path—known as Bowl Loop—circling the huge grassy hollow. As you go, pause periodically to admire the fine city views off to your right.

At the opposite side of the bowl, if you want to continue this walk on flat ground, complete the Bowl Loop, circle back to where you started, and return down the slope toward the artificial stream and lake.

Otherwise, bear right onto a smaller path known as Diane's Trail, and follow this downhill through bunches of cactus.

Keep to the right as the trail winds along and goes through a series of switchbacks, gradually climbing to a plateau. As you go, you'll have more opportunities to appreciate what these hills would look like without the park—oil derricks, pumping crude oil out of the dry, dusty hills.

As the trail flattens, continue walking straight ahead through a grove of low-growing California pepper trees and then a grove of eucalyptus, heading for a shaded rest area at the trail's apex.

This is Autumn's Peak, and the views are spectacular. Around you is a sweeping panorama, offering uninterrupted views of Palos Verdes, LAX, and Catalina to the south, Marina Del Rey, Santa Monica, and Point Dume to the west, Beverly Hills, Westwood, Century City, the Miracle Mile, and Hollywood to the north, and downtown L.A., Mount Baldy, and the San Gabriel Mountains to the east.

You can pick out the landmarks: the old and new control towers at LAX; the buildings of Ocean Avenue in Santa Monica; the Mormon Church's white spire in lower Westwood; the twin towers of Century City; the bright blue and green blocks of West Hollywood's Pacific Design Center; and the Hollywood Sign and the Griffith Park Observatory, high above.

When you have sufficiently feasted your eyes and captured enough images for Instagram, head downhill, following the wide path as it approaches another shaded rest area—this one named Christine's Point.

Just before you arrive there, though, veer right onto a much narrower path. Follow this downhill through a series of switchbacks until you come to a T-intersection.

Turn left onto a flat trail bordered by a steep slope on the left, and wind downhill a little more, dropping in time down a flight of concrete steps to land at Randi's Waterfall.

This is another faux water feature, featuring a stream, a pond, and some falling water, that on a hot day can be very refreshing, and even tempting. Swimming, though, is discouraged.

Instead, walk on, under one red torii gate, and then another, to find the final hidden secret of this park.

This is Doris's Japanese Garden, a pair of lotus-covered ponds connected by curved bridges and landscaped in the Japanese style. It's not as nice or as ornate as the Japanese Garden near the water treatment plant in the Sepulveda Basin (for that, see Walk #29), but it's pretty good, considering what this area would look like otherwise.

Leave the garden through a large gate protected by stone lions, and walk straight ahead through a parking lot. When you see the parking kiosk ahead, cross the main road and find the paved sidewalk. Turn left, going uphill slightly, to return to your parking place.

220

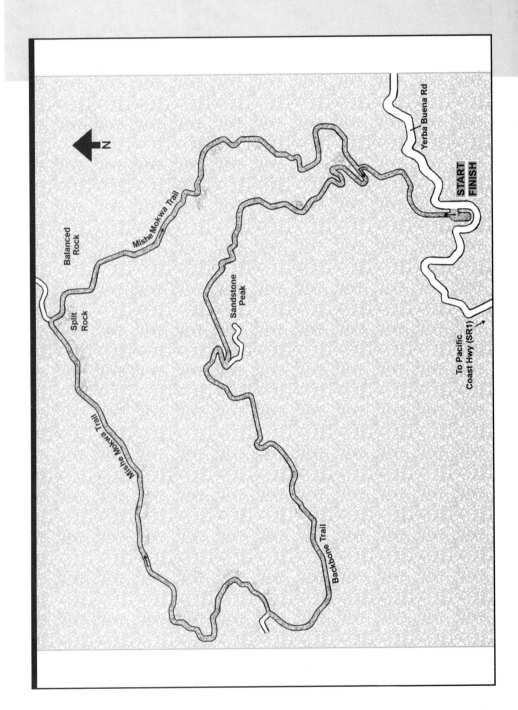

WALK #41

SANDSTONE PEAK
DISTANCE: **6 miles**
DURATION: **3–4 hours**
DIFFICULTY: **5**
DETAILS: **Free parking.**
Dogs on leash allowed.

The longest walk in this collection, and the most challenging, this is a glorious, hilly hike across varied terrain that in places is reminiscent of Sedona or Moab, but with vast ocean and city views. Best in cool, dry weather and not recommended on a very hot or rainy day, it has a great picnic spot at its center point.

Begin this walk high in the Santa Monica Mountains. Leave the Pacific Coast Highway (SR 1) on Yerba Buena Road, then drive about six miles (just past Circle X Ranch) to find the Sandstone Peak parking lot

If you're coming from the Valley, take Westlake Boulevard off the 101, follow it until it becomes Decker Canyon, turn right where Decker merges with Mulholland Highway, and then turn right onto Little Sycamore Canyon Road. This becomes Yerba Buena. The parking area is 4.5 miles from the turn off at Mulholland.

Find the trail leading from the parking lot, going uphill. Watch for a split in this path and bear left onto Backbone Trail, headed for Sandstone Peak. (You can take a more direct and difficult route by turning right onto the Mishe Mokwa Trail, which is a shorter and much more arduous hike.)

Heading uphill, you'll find the going pretty steep. The good news: it doesn't last long, and it's the hardest part of the walk.

Already the views are good, particularly of Sandstone Peak itself, which at 3,111 feet is the highest point in the Santa Monica Mountain Range.

Walk on, as the trail winds through scrub oak and chaparral. At the crest, take a spur trail to the top of Sandstone for breathtaking views of the Pacific. Then continue along the Backbone Trail.

The trail will drop through a red-rock area and then into some areas shaded by brush, before flattening into a very gradual descent into a wooded canyon. Here views switch from ocean and mountain to valley floor, with looks at Thousand Oaks and Westlake Village.

Where the trail splits again, take the Mishe Mokwa Trail on the right for Split Rock—not the Backbone Trail, heading for Tri Peaks. (That is part of the great ridge trail that runs from Will Rogers Historic State Park all the way north to about Oxnard. For more information, see Walk #35.)

The trail will eventually wind around and deposit you at Split Rock, a picturesque picnic area divided by a flowing creek and named after a set of huge, cracked boulders standing beside the trail. There is ample shade here for a cool, quiet rest before starting back on the return journey.

You have two choices for the walk back: you can go back the way you came and dig some more of those massive ocean views going downhill, or you can walk across the shady picnic area and continue on the Mishe Mokwa Trail, which crosses the creek and climbs steeply up to the left and out of the Split Rock area.

The posted signs say it's 1.7 miles back to the parking area—and it's a real hike, with sections that are quite demanding.

It's also quite rewarding, though. The trail climbs out of the canyon, hugging the sheer sandstone walls where rock climbers gather to practice their craft.

Near them is Balanced Rock, and far beyond that, you can see Malibu Lake.

The terrain gradually becomes drier as the trail crests and begins to descend. You'll see a trail that looks like it's headed for a parking lot below. That's the rock climbers' parking lot, though—not yours.

Pass this by, and continue until you meet the intersection you crossed at the beginning of the walk. Bear left and head downhill for the last section of this walk. At the bottom of the trail, you will be back at your starting point.

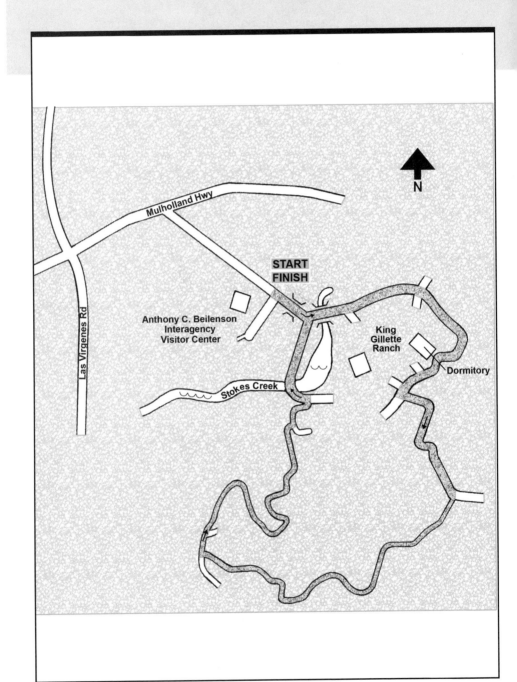

WALK #42

KING GILLETTE RANCH
  DISTANCE: **1.5 miles**
  DURATION: **40 minutes**
  DIFFICULTY: **2**
  DETAILS: **Park open from 7 am to sunset. Free two-hour parking. Wheelchair accessible from Visitor Center to ranch buildings. No dogs allowed.**

Here's a short, gentle hike through a northern piece of the Santa Monica Mountains and around the grounds of a great historic home—once the playground of high-society Hollywood personalities. To make this walk a little longer, and tougher, follow the signs in the middle of the walk for "Inspiration Point," a side trip that will add about fifteen minutes to the whole hike.

Begin your walk in the Malibu Hills, just east of the intersection of Mulholland Highway and Las Virgenes Road—not far from the entrance to Malibu Creek State Park, which also offers some good walking and is popular with hikers.

Enter the King Gillette Ranch property off Mulholland, turning in at a long driveway shadowed by eucalyptus trees. Drive past the little guard shack at the top of this long lane. Then turn right at the first opportunity, into the parking lot for the Anthony C. Beilenson Interagency Visitor Center.

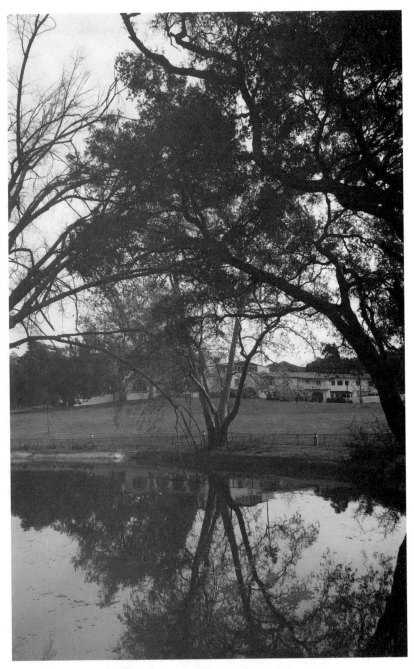

A peaceful pond near the Gillette home.

Park here and, before setting out, take advantage of the restrooms and (on some weekend days) a table with big canisters of cold drinking water. Then go back to the driveway, turn right, and begin walking.

Cross a bridge and turn left at the T-intersection. Then cross another bridge, walking in the direction of signs that say "Parking." Then bear right and continue up the driveway, in the direction marked "Resident Parking Only." Walk straight on, headed for an archway in the big, white Spanish-style building ahead of you. Cross through the arch and bear left.

Some distance ahead is another large, white Spanish-style building. Walk toward that, keeping to the left, and soak up some history.

King Gillette—whose full given name was King Camp Gillette—was the fellow who first mastered the mass production of cheap, disposable razor blades. He became extremely wealthy and spent some of his energy concocting plans for a great utopian socialist state. He spent some of his money on real estate.

Gillette purchased a large tract of land where you are now walking, and hired popular Los Angeles architect Wallace Neff (best known for designing Pickfair, the estate of Hollywood lovebirds Mary Pickford and Douglas Fairbanks) to build a rambling home in his signature Spanish Colonial Revival style.

Gillette split his time between here and Palm Springs, until his death in 1932. The property was then acquired by the MGM director Clarence Brown, who specialized in Joan Crawford and Greta Garbo pictures. Brown had an airstrip built, it is said, in order to fly in Hollywood friends for lavish parties. Bob Hope later owned the property, but gave it to the Claretian order of the Catholic Church, which established a seminary here.

The Claretians built the three-story building on your left as the dormitory, which performed the same function for subsequent owners. Those included Elizabeth Clare Prophet, who ran her Church Universal and Triumphant from here for a time, and Soka University of America, the local branch of an educational institution founded by the Soka Gakkai Buddhist organization in Japan. After Soka decamped for Orange County, the land was taken over by the state and became a 588-acre public park in 2005. In 2020, the building stood in for fictional Lucia State Hospital in the Netflix series *Ratched*.

Walk on past this dormitory and a line of nicely tended rose bushes. Go straight ahead, toward another low, white period building. Walk with this on your left until the pavement ends, marked by a sign saying it's open to authorized vehicles only, and you are on a dirt road bordering an open dirt field. Walk on a bit and, just to your right, find a narrow path rising slightly into oaky shade.

This path, dotted with horse tracks and horse droppings, will wander around the edge of a hill, then meet a paved road. Turn right onto the road and take it to the crest of a slight hill, then turn right onto a dirt trail that narrows as it wends downhill past some incongruous overhead lighting.

The path descends into good shade, then merges with a paved road. Walk straight ahead, ignoring a paved road to the left, to a Y-intersection. Bear left, and when you meet another Y-intersection just after, do the same.

You'll see a picnic table here, a good place for a snack. You might also see a workout area over to the right, and some people grunting and sweating there. Don't be alarmed. These are contestants on the TV show *The Biggest Loser*, which has its base camp, and does some of its filming, in the surrounding area. As you walk along, the next building on your left may have a sign over its door indicating as much.

The road will bend left in front of another low, white building of somewhat more recent construction, which is a new dormitory for the "Losers." Just after this, near a sign reading "No Roadside Parking," turn right and cross the lawn toward a small body of water at the bottom of the hill.

Here you will find ducks, the shade of big sycamore trees, lush grass, and the best views of the Gillette home. The pond is part of Stokes Creek, and is said to be home to cormorant, heron, and other water birds, though I have only seen mallards on the water here.

When you've soaked up enough shade and architecture, walk straight along the water until you meet the paved road once more. Turn left and cross the bridge, then bear right, cross another bridge, and you'll be back at the visitor center and your starting place.

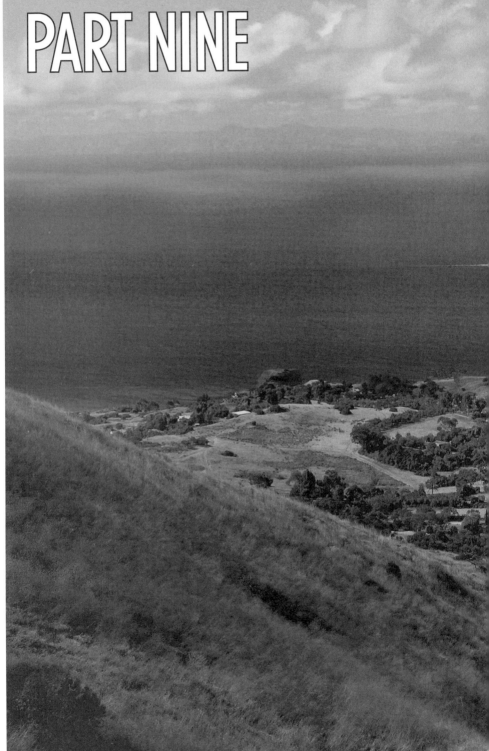

PART NINE

SOUTH BAY

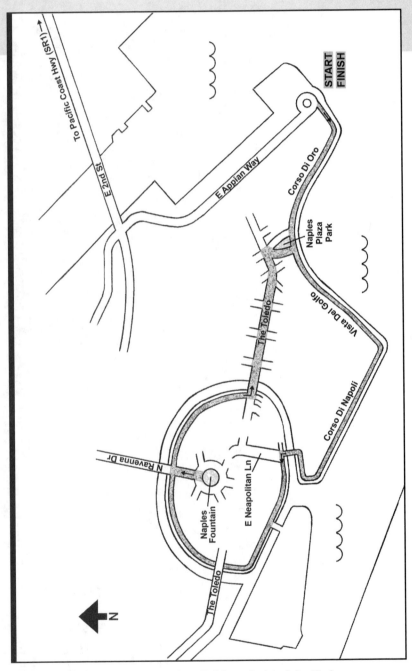

Overleaf: A view of the Pacific Ocean from Del Cerro Park in Palos Verdes.

WALK #43

THE NAPLES CANALS
DISTANCE: **2.2 miles**
DURATION: **1 hour**
DIFFICULTY: **2**
DETAILS: **Free street parking.**
Dogs on leash allowed.
Long Beach Transit bus #131.

This is the southern sister of the Venice Canals—another net-work of waterways interlaced with houses that offers great walking. It's especially good on a hot day, when it's nice to be close to the water, or at Christmas, when the community hosts a parade of its decorated boats.

Start your walk in Long Beach near the intersection of Second Street and Pacific Coast Highway (SR 1), at the southern end of East Appian Way.

Park on the street (or get off the bus) as close as possible to the cul-de-sac end of Appian, near the Long Beach Yacht Club. Then, with Appian behind you, the yacht club on your left, and the wide canal directly before you, turn right and begin strolling down the sidewalk known as Corso di Oro.

This whole construction sprang from the fevered imagination of land speculator Arthur Parson, in partnership with the railroad magnate Henry Huntington. Inspired by Venice's developer Abbot Kinney, in the early 1900s Parson began dredging and digging a section of Alamitos Bay in the mouth of the San Gabriel River to build a place where, as he conceived it, "through the canals and under the high arching bridges gay gondoliers will propel their crafts like those in the waters of the Adriatic under the blue skies of Italy."

He called it the "Dreamland of Southern California."

It took decades for the project to be realized, and then took years for much of it to be rebuilt after the massive 6.4-magnitude earthquake destroyed much of Long Beach in 1933.

The street names reflect Parson's Italian reverie. As you follow the sidewalk, keeping the water on your left, you'll move from Corso di Oro to Vista del Golfo to Corso di Napoli.

Stay on the sidewalk as it bends right, toward the central island of the Naples Canal. Then take the first left, up and over the East Neapolitan Lane bridge.

From the bridge, you may see kayakers, or even gondoliers. Though they may not be the colorful, gay Neapolitan variety, the gondolas are available to rent by the hour for romantic visits of the canals.

On the other side of the water, turn left and return to the sidewalk running along the water. This is the Rivo Alto Canal.

Follow the waterway, keeping the canal on your left, and enjoy a leisurely stroll. You'll pass many elegant homes with well-manicured lawns and gardens. These homes get extremely dressed up for the holidays, too, as if competing with the decorated boats that participate in the canal parade.

As you go, you'll cross several roadways, using the steps provided to go up and over them. These all have Italian-inspired names, too, or names borrowed directly from Italian cities—Siena, Venetia, Tivoli, Via di Roma, and Garibaldi being only a few.

The first big intersection you meet will be at a street known as the Toledo. Cross this and continue walking along another charming stretch of canal, fronted by well-maintained homes.

Soon you'll come to another big intersection, this one called North Ravenna Drive. Here, you'll take a detour: at the roadway, turn right and walk two blocks into the very heart of Naples, to the large fountain surrounded by a park that is the core of this fabulous, fabricated island.

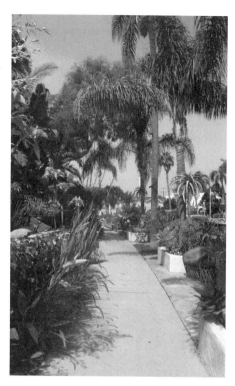

The Naples sidewalks are nicely landscaped by the homeowners whose houses face the canal.

When you've tossed a coin and made a wish, return along Ravenna to the Rivo Alto Canal Walk, turn right, and continue your clockwise circumnavigation of the island.

When you meet the next major intersection—the Toledo, again—turn left and go up and over the canal. Follow this road past narrow streets called Via di Roma, Savona, Angelo, and Giralda. It will then lead you slightly to the left until you arrive at a small bit of greenery known as Naples Plaza Park.

Turn right here, and walk toward the water. You will soon find your original Corso di Oro sidewalk by the water, with great views of the canal going into Alamitos Bay.

Turn left along the Corso, and walk the quarter mile or so back to the bottom of Appian Way, where you'll find your starting point.

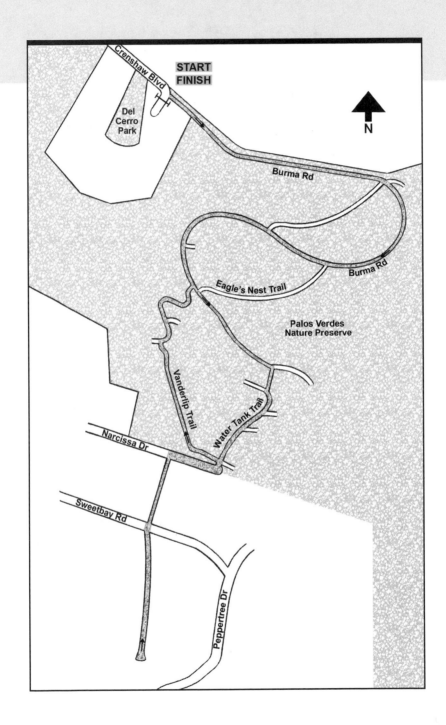

WALK #44

DEL CERRO PARK
DISTANCE: **4 miles**
DURATION: **1 hour 30 minutes to 2 hours**
DIFFICULTY: **4**
DETAILS: **Free street parking.**
Dogs on leash allowed.

This walk is pretty far from home for a lot of Angelenos, but it's such a great spot that it's worth a little drive just for the spectacular ocean views. To make a half-day of it, do this walk, then drive down to the little public walking trail at Trump National Golf Club for lunch and a stroll on the beach. To get good parking, get there early.

Begin this walk at the very southern end of Crenshaw Boulevard, west of the Harbor Freeway (I-110) and south of the Pacific Coast Highway (SR 1), where Crenshaw climbs up into the hills and stops at a wide metal gate.

Park your car where Crenshaw meets Burrell Lane—or as close to that as possible—and walk past the metal gate. Though it isn't marked as such, this is the Burma Road trail entrance to the Palos Verdes Nature Preserve. It begins as a wide dirt road, passing between some houses before opening up onto some fine vistas.

You may see Catalina Island from here. You will certainly see the blue Pacific Ocean and the Portuguese Bend area of the Palos Verdes coastline, as you descend gradually past pepper trees and clumps of cactus, sage, and wild mustard.

After half a mile or so of gentle descent, the Burma Road trail will sweep wide and to the right. (There is a large water storage tank here, and a public portable toilet.) After the sweep, take the Eagles Nest spur trail off to the left, and walk toward the stand of pine trees for some superior beach views. Then return to the broad Burma dirt road and continue as it descends and swings left.

Here, you may hear some birds squawking. This noise is coming from some of the locals—peacocks and peahens, which make a sharp "kee-yaw" sound that echoes through the canyon.

The local historians say that the birds arrived here in the form of a gift. An early Palos Verdes developer, Frank Vanderlip, who served in President William McKinley's cabinet in the last decade of the 1800s, received the peafowl from William Wrigley, the owner of the famous chewing gum company. (He also owned the Chicago Cubs and Catalina Island.)

Vanderlip was a visionary. He had come to the area to recover from an illness, and was so taken by the scenery that he negotiated the purchase of twenty-five square miles of open land. He commissioned Frederick Law Olmsted and John Charles Olmsted (who designed New York's Central Park and San Francisco's Golden Gate Park) to lay out streets and parks for a seaside suburb community. This is what eventually became Palos Verdes Estates; however, the area you're enjoying now was never developed.

This Burma Road trail continues for quite a distance, all the way across this nature preserve to approximately the end of Portuguese Bend Road, ultimately connecting to streets and houses again. However, on this walk you're going to take a detour that will lead more directly to a cliff with some fine ocean views.

On your right, you'll find a steep, straight trail known as the Water Tank Trail, shortcutting some of the distance out of the descent. Take this trail—carefully, especially if the ground is wet or slippery—and walk straight down until you meet a paved road—the cul-de-sac end of Narcissa Drive.

Turn right onto Narcissa, and walk about 100 feet. On your

left, you'll see a wide, bare field with a path running across it. Take this path straight ahead, until it rises to a bluff sitting high over the beaches at Portuguese Bend, Smugglers Cove, and Abalone Cove.

After you've soaked up the view and prepared yourself for the walk back, return to Narcissa the way you came. Turn right onto the paved road, and walk toward the cul-de-sac end. Turn left, as if you were going to walk the Water Tank Trail, up the steep incline.

But instead of doing that, take a narrow trail—known locally as Vanderlip Trail—heading off to the left. Enjoy this gradual climb through low-growing wild mustard, wheat, and fennel. The trail will run fairly straight, then eventually bend right and get a little steeper. When you hit a wide, dirt road, turn left.

You're back on the Burma Road trail, above the spot where you turned off onto the steep Water Tank Trail. Follow the Burma Road trail back the way you came, making a gradual ascent. The road will get steeper, but the views will get better, too. As you tire, take a break and turn around for some splendid scenery.

When the dirt road meets paved road again, you are back on Crenshaw, and back at your starting point.

ACKNOWLEDGMENTS

I would not have written this book had it not been for the support of Julie Singer, and could not have written it without the help of Jeffrey Goldman, Kate Murray, and Bryan Duddles.

I also received good counsel and guidance on L.A. and walking from my L.A. Walks column editors Alice Short and Mary MacVean.

I would also like to thank the following walking enthusiasts, who were kind enough to test these walks and share their experiences: J.T. Allen, Teri Aranguen, Arlene Bernstein, Linda Beaumaster, Sally Beddon, Jill Brown, Priscilla Brown, Jon Burk, Vincent Castellanos, Erika Chaumontet, Sandi Cochran, Johann and Joane Diel, Lisa Dupuy, Erik Ekstrand, Ruth Eliel, Elena Estrin, Sam and Paige Farmer, Anya Farquhar, Tara Fass, John Ferdenzi, Mauricio Figuls, Steve Finkel, Margaret Gatz, Laura Geffen, Tim Gibbons, Marcia Gimbrone, Roger Hatchett, Kate Hawkes, Eleanor Heaphy, Carol Henning, Karen Howard, Holly Huckins, Phil Jamtaas, Leah Kabaker, Shawn Kelly, Jan Keizer, David Kipen, Mitchell Landsberg, Geoff Larsen, Maya Levinson, Roni Long, Evelyn Mah, Chris Martins, Mary MacVean, April Mundy, Kim Nagele, Richard Natale, Katherine Nilbrink, Mark Parra, Marino Pascal, Gayle Penrod, Claudia Peschiutta, Kenneth Robbins, Dave and Kama Rowley, Ellen Slezak, Terry Solis, Chris Spicher, Kathy Sturdevant, Sandra Tapia, Bonnie Thompson, Monk Turner, Stephanie Vendig, Scott Wardlaw, Bill Weidner, Regina West, Stephen Williams, and Dan Wolf.